Acquiring Competency and Achieving Proficiency with

DIALECTICAL BEHAVIOR THERAPY

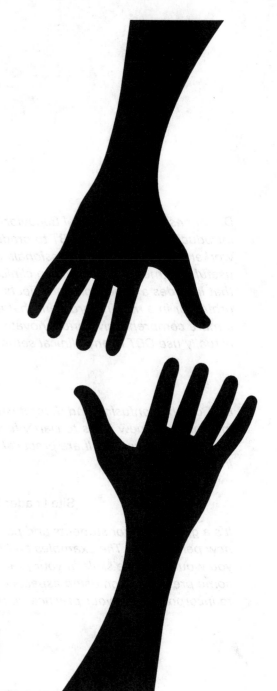

Volume I
The Clinician's Guidebook

Cathy Moonshine, Ph.D., MAC, CADC III

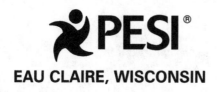

PESI®

EAU CLAIRE, WISCONSIN

D1291477

Dr. Moonshine's Dialectical Behavior Therapy Guidebook for Clinicians is the ideal tool for introducing "real world" DBT to graduate students, psychologists, psychiatrists, social workers and all health professionals who want to review new applications of an extremely useful treatment. Her extensive clinical experience with DBT is evident in this practical text that includes a variety of worksheets that clinicians can readily integrate into their work. As a professor in a training program that emphasizes evidence-based treatment, I cannot imagine a more comprehensive and innovative teaching tool for training my students in how to actually use DBT in any clinical setting.

Michael Christopher, PhD
Assistant Professor @ School of Professional Psychology

DBT can be confusing and theoretical. Dr. Moonshine puts her unique slant on it, incorporating new ideas to clarify fundamental DBT concepts. These volume as well as the worksheets in volume II are practical and help the counselor and client develop competence in the skills.

Emily Hedges, M.A., CADC III
Site Leader @ Western Psychological Services & Counseling Services

It's a great book for students and people who want to learn DBT or for those who just want a new perspective. The examples and handouts make it very easy to apply to clients or see how you would use the skills in your practice. It's really easy to understand and helped clarify some previously confusing aspects of DBT. This book presents DBT as very flexible and easy to incorporate into your practice no matter what your orientation.

Dean Charles, M.S.
Counselor @ Springbrook Hazelton

"Got to make it somehow on the dreams you still believe."

To MH for riding along with me on the rollercoaster of my wacky ideas, outlandish plans and off the wall projects.

To VH for teaching me so much and pushing me to learn more.

To my mentors and colleagues for sharing their perspective and experience.

To my past, present and future students, supervisees and mentees for being committed to professional growth while maintaining a sense of humor.

For clients everywhere to find their path.

Copyright © 2008 PESI, LLC

PESI, LLC
PO Box 1000
3839 White Avenue
Eau Claire, Wisconsin 54702

Printed in the United States of America

ISBN: 978-0-9790218-4-8

PESI, LLC strives to obtain knowledgeable authors and faculty for its publications and seminars. The clinical recommendations contained herein are the result of extensive author research and review. Obviously, any recommendations for patient care must be held up against individual circumstances at hand. To the best of our knowledge any recommendations included by the author or faculty reflect currently accepted practice. However, these recommendations cannot be considered universal and complete. The authors and publisher repudiate any responsibility for unfavorable effects that result from information, recommendations, undetected omissions or errors. Professionals using this publication should research other original sources of authority as well.

For information on this and other PESI manuals and
audio recordings, please call 800-843-7763 or
visit our website at www.pesi.com

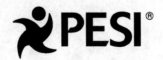

Table of Contents

About the Author

Cathy Moonshine, PhD, MAC, CADC III is the Executive Director of a private consulting firm, Moonshine Consulting as well as assistant professor at the School of Professional Psychology at Pacific University in Portland, Oregon. Dr. Moonshine is an expert trainer, clinical supervisor and clinician. In 2007, Dr. Moonshine created and published DBT board game, playing cards, bingo, and bonanza dice game. All of these and other resources are available at the D.B.T. in Life™ Store at http://www.Moonshine-Consulting.com.

Dr. Moonshine is largely self-taught in Dialectic Behavior Therapy ("DBT"). She has read many books and professional articles on DBT and has utilized clinical supervision and consultation with colleagues to increase her competency with this model. Dr. Moonshine completed her doctoral education at Pacific Graduate School of Psychology in Palo Alto, CA. She received her Master's from Seattle University and Bachelor's from University of Redlands.

Dr. Moonshine has modified DBT to work with clients, graduate students, supervisees, and in program oversight. Dr. Moonshine focuses on balancing dialectics, being mindfully present, and making use of DBT skills. The DBT skills that Dr. Moonshine utilizes in her work include ones originally created by Dr. Marsha Linehan and/or other authors. Dr. Moonshine has sought to utilize the most successful aspects of the traditional DBT model in combination with her own successful treatment philosophies, patient methods, and teaching skills.

Dr. Moonshine acknowledges with gratitude Dr. Linehan as the creator of the DBT model. However, all trainings, clinical support, and products created or sold by Dr. Moonshine are of her own creation without collaboration with Dr. Linehan, or Dr. Linehan's affiliated company, Behavioral Tech, LLC. Dr. Moonshine's products are not sanctioned by, sponsored, licensed, or affiliated with Dr. Linehan and/or Behavioral Tech, LLC. Clinicians and programs interested in providing full fidelity to the empirically supported DBT protocol and wishing to be recognized as official DBT clinicians should contact Behavioral Tech at http://www.behavioraltech.org or (206) 675-8588.

Dr. Moonshine has over twenty years of experience in public and private mental health and substance abuse treatment settings across all levels of care. Dr. Moonshine provides licensure supervision and collegial consultation to mental health, addictions and dual diagnosis clinicians. She works with systems of care and individual clinicians to implement and sustain evidenced based practices. Dr. Moonshine serves as Clinical Director for nearly 10 years in Portland, Oregon. In addition to Clinical Director duties, Dr. Moonshine continues to make an impact in the local, state and national treatment communities with her consultation, supervision and trainings. Dr. Moonshine is considered an expert in the areas of addictions and dual diagnosis treatment.

CHAPTER 1
Introduction

HOW IT ALL BEGAN

Dialectical Behavior Therapy, also known as DBT, has been gaining the interest of researchers, clinicians, and clients for nearly 15 years. The original text and skills manual were published in 1993, although there were a number of peer review articles published in professional journals prior to this date (Linehan 1993a; Linehan 1993b). Today, there are over 400 articles and many books that have been published on this topic (See PsycINFO). The popularity of DBT can be attributed to its demonstrated success with high-need, challenging clients.

DBT was created by Marsha Linehan, Ph.D., and was originally designed to address the needs of chronically suicidal clients for whom the models in use at that time were insufficient (Linehan 1993a; Linehan 1993b). In many communities there were dozens—perhaps hundreds—of chronically suicidal clients over-utilizing acute care resources such as emergency rooms and inpatient hospital beds. No matter what therapy some of these clients received or psychiatric medications they took, their lives were filled with self-hatred and despair.

Families and other support networks engaged in various strategies to assist their loved ones. Treatment professionals were at a loss as to how to adequately treat these clients so that they could live independently and with some life satisfaction. Many professionals dedicated themselves to finding clinical methods or biological interventions that would meet the clients' needs. For some clients, this resulted in relief of symptoms, remission, and perhaps even recovery from their mental health and substance use difficulties. For many other clients, it felt like one failure after another. If their therapists, psychologists, psychiatric nurse practitioners, psychiatrists, and medical doctors couldn't collaborate with their friends and families to find a cure, then the client felt hopeless and believed that life wasn't worth living.

Treatment professionals from various backgrounds also believed that it might be hopeless. Self-doubt and fears of incompetence plagued many professionals. Some professionals chose not to work with these clients. In the worst-case scenarios, professionals acted out their own countertransference and negative emotional reactions by firing clients, becoming angry or immobilized, withdrawing, and finding other ways of disengaging from these clients.

Along came DBT. Investigation revealed that many of these chronically suicidal clients, whom it was originally designed to treat, qualified for a diagnosis of Borderline Personality Disorder (BPD). Over the last two decades many research studies have supported the effectiveness of the Dialectical Behavior Therapy approach with BPD. More recently DBT has been demonstrated to be effective with other clinical presentations, both in research protocols and with anecdotal evidence.

THEORY, PHILOSOPHY, AND MAJOR GOAL

INTERNAL EXPERIENCES

DBT is based on the theory that clients have internal distress. Clients are emotionally intuitive and sensitive and, as a survival mechanism, many clients have learned to pick up on how others feel about them. While this can be inaccurate, it is close enough to reality for clients to engage in control behavior based on their assessments of how people feel about them. Clients use this ability to manage their relationships and behaviors.

This is particularly important in the therapeutic relationship. It is essential that clinicians are able to form genuine empathic relationships with appropriate boundaries. This last statement is an example of dialectic: it is a "both/and" statement, as opposed to an "either/or" statement. Both sides of the dialectic are important: the empathic relationships and the boundaries. Clients will sense how their clinicians feel about them so it is particularly important that clinicians maintain a balance with this dialectic.

Clinicians also have an ethical responsibility to manage their feelings towards clients; either excessively positive or excessively negative feelings can be problematic. Some models refer to this as countertransference. Clinicians can maintain balance in the therapeutic relationship and manage their countertransference issues by being mindful of both positive and negative feelings and reactions. This mindfulness facilitates processing of the countertransference with supervisors or peers to adequately diffuse strong emotions.

Being emotionally intense and slow to return to baseline are two internal experiences common to many clients. These clients feel their emotions more intensely than the typical person. Instead of rating an emotion on a scale from one to ten, these clients' emotions are off the chart. A one-to-ten scale doesn't give them enough range—their experience is often an 11, 15 or 100. Their feelings are very intense most of the time. Additionally, these same clients may feel their emotions for an extended amount of time. While it takes typical people 30 to 45 minutes to return to their baseline emotional state, these clients might take hours, days, or as much as a week to return to their baseline emotional state.

Clinicians now realize that these clients have internal experiences that are different from those of the average person. Their internal experience is more intense, chaotic, and troublesome than the typical person's. These clients benefit from the here-and-now perspective, frustration tolerance, emotional regulation, and effectiveness in relationships skills provided by adopting a DBT perspective and using these skills in their lives.

EXTERNAL EXPERIENCES

If the client's internal experience is as described above, then these individuals may have different experiences in their relationships and environments than the average person as well. According to DBT theory, these individuals hear from family and friends that the ways they think, communicate, and behave is inappropriate, unacceptable, and wrong. They must think, communicate, and behave in different ways. This is invalidating. Clients are told to be completely different from their true selves, which is highly unlikely if not impossible.

Another frequent experience is punishment or abuse when the client displays painful emotions and problematic behaviors. Both children and adults sometimes act out their emotional experiences. They lose control of their tempers or are inconsolably sad or upset. They may behave in problematic ways by getting into physical fights, harming themselves, drinking, using drugs, engaging in out-of-control eating, dangerous sexual encounters, gambling, or spending excessively, to name just a few examples. They reject help and don't think anything can help them manage their emotions more effectively. There may be an attitude of self-righteousness or hopelessness in their defense of their emotions or behaviors. Their emotions and behaviors can result in punishment or abuse by others who label them as excessive and over-the-top.

Additionally, these clients hear from family and friends that their problems are not that bad and that they could find solutions a lot more easily if they just tried. To illustrate this point here are some examples of what clients have heard:

- "Stop being such a drama queen."
- "Just get over it."
- "Pull yourself up."
- "Stop making it worse than it needs to be."
- "You want something to cry about, I'll give you something to cry about."
- "You think you have it bad, I had it worse."
- "Why aren't you more like…"
- "You need to be less like . . ."

CUMULATIVE EFFECT OF INTERNAL AND EXTERNAL EXPERIENCES

If the clients have the internal and external experiences outlined above, then it makes sense that they are who they are. If these things happened once or twice it probably wouldn't result in their current problems, but as a chronic and entrenched experience it disrupts normal development. They have experienced disrespect, disappointment, and trauma again and again. They have been unable to effectively tap into their skills, strengths, and resiliency. It is logical that these clients will benefit from therapy and that DBT skills can provide the essential building blocks to rebuild their lives into those worth living (Linehan 1993a; Linehan 1993b).

PHILOSOPHY

There are two major philosophical points in DBT:

1. *Clients are doing the best they can and need better skills to be more effective.*

Given the internal and external experiences of these clients, it is easy to understand their behavior. They are highly sensitive, emotionally intense, and slow to return to baseline. Because they find themselves living in invalidating environments with people who take advantage of them, abuse and punish them, it only makes sense that they would engage in problematic, destructive behaviors. Anyone with the same internal strengths and weaknesses, the same external experiences and life trajectory, would no doubt exhibit similar or worse tendencies. These clients are doing the best the can with what they've got. DBT provides a place of compassion and understanding for these clients. This is a useful stance for both the clinician and client to have, but it is only half the story. The other side of this dialectic is that clients have to work hard, learn their DBT skills, and use them in their daily lives. The both/and perspective is that the clients are doing the best they can with what they've got and they absolutely have to work hard by using DBT skills to be more effective in their lives. Clinicians are encouraged to maintain the optimal balance with this philosophical point.

The following is an example of how a clinician would use this dialectic: a client comes into treatment and reports wanting his life to be better. The client engages in near daily non-lethal self-harm behaviors of cutting and burning. Over the first two months of therapy the clinician teaches assertiveness skills, illustrates the importance of self-care, and focuses on the reduction of depression. The client is still using self-harm as way to deal with stress. The clinician is frustrated and feels hopeless because the client won't change this highly problematic behavior. The forward momentum seems to stop and there is a lot of tension in the room between the clinician and the client.

If the clinician can apply the philosophy that the client is doing the best he can and needs to learn DBT skills to be more effective in his life, this situation can be resolved. The first half of this dialectic requires both the clinician and client to realize and accept that the client's behavior serves a function. It relieves stress, provides familiarity, and perhaps confirms the client's negative self-judgment. The behavior was very useful in the client's chaotic and abusive family during his formative years. The client has used this behavior to feel grounded, alive, and in control of something. It makes sense given the client's history that this would be a reasonable behavior for awhile. This is a stance of compassion and understanding that is very useful to the clinician, the client, and the therapeutic relationship but it is only half the story.

The other half of the story comes after the clinician validates the client and the clinician then requires him to stop the self-harm behavior. The clinician explains that the goal of DBT is to build a life worth living (Linehan 1993a; Linehan 1993b). Continued self-harm or other destructive behaviors run contrary to this goal. While it may not be easier for the client to stop the self-harm behavior (otherwise the client would have already done that) it is absolutely essential. At this point the clinician selects DBT skills that will help meet the needs the self-harm behavior fulfilled to replace the need for self-harm behavior. Some suggested skills for this might be **Non-Judgmental, Radical Acceptance, MEDDSS, FAST, or Ride the Wave.** The client will learn and practice the skills. Slips and relapse of self-harm behavior will be dealt with and recommitment to using the skills and not harming the self will be very useful techniques. Ultimately the client dedicates himself to being as effective as he can be which requires finding more effective ways to deal with stress.

2. *Clients have not caused all their problems but they have to solve them anyway.*

This is true for everyone in the world. There are times when individuals create or contribute to their own problems, while there are other times when problems simply happen. This philosophical perspective gets clients out of the victim or martyr stance even when they have terrible things in their history and empowers them to be effective in the here and now.

Clients who get stuck in the mindset that things "shouldn't" have happened to them may feel the need to process excessively in hopes of making sense of or understanding their negative experiences. Some clients believe that if they can find a reason, or make sense of it, it won't be so bad. Unfortunately, whatever has happened, whether in the recent or distant past, can't be changed and focusing on it excessively is unproductive. Spending excessive time reflecting on the past can get in the way of living right now.

A clinical example of this situation is a client who was raped or sexually molested. They spend years in therapy trying to figure out what they did wrong, how they asked for it or wondering if they enjoyed it. Most of their time, energy, and attention are spent reliving the past with hopes of finding meaning in it. This client is trying to say "This happened to me for a reason." Well, sometimes bad things happen to people for no apparent reason. Sometimes clients put themselves in harm's way but they didn't ask for it or enjoy it in any way. This philosophical point supports clients in acknowledging the trauma, productively learning from it, and resolving any issues before moving back to living the majority of their lives in the here and now.

This DBT philosophy is also useful when clients have a faulty belief that if something is unfair then it shouldn't apply to them. They have a political, ethical, or legal perspective that things shouldn't be the way they are and hence they should not have to comply with that requirement. Things a client might say that are indicative of this faulty belief include:

- "Marijuana should be legal so I'm gonna smoke it."
- "Corporations are ripping people off so I can steal things from them."

- "It's not fair so I am just going to do what I want."
- "My parents abused me, so what if I do hurt people physically. It happened to me so it can happen to them."
- "My life sucks so I am making it painful for others."

These clients can discuss for hours how their perspective applies to them because things shouldn't have happened or that reality should be different than it is. There may even be a kernel of truth or reality in their viewpoint but the entitlement that these clients bring to their perspective is ineffective. There are many things in life that are unfair. Sometimes people don't get what they want. That does not mean that they should not be held responsible for their behavior or expected to act appropriately. Ultimately, clients haven't always caused their problems, but they have to solve them anyway and deal with any aftermath that ensues.

SYNTHESIS OF INTERNAL AND EXTERNAL CAUSES

According to DBT clinical symptoms, problems, and distress result from disconnections and stress between the individual and his surroundings. Clients may not be able to read clues or understand expectations in certain roles or situations. They may have difficulty meeting opposing needs, which tend to be dialectics. For example, a common dialectic is the desire to be independent and self-sufficient while also wanting to be in a relationship and be taken care of sometimes. Another dialectic would be simultaneous fear of, and desire for, success.

These clients have histories of problematic attachment, trauma, significant loss and genetic predisposition to mental health difficulties. They will experience more balance when they can cope emotionally and stay focused on solutions. Balance will also be facilitated when clients can develop the ability to process internal and external information. Another useful component for clients is the ability to be grounded right now while being connected with the near and distant future. Clients can learn to balance their feelings and behaviors as well as threats and safety effectively. All of these dialectics can be balanced through DBT treatment and using DBT skills in daily life.

THERAPY-INTERFERING BEHAVIORS

Therapy-interfering behaviors are things that get in the way of the therapy or treatment. This is a two-way street to which both clients and clinicians contribute. Clients and families do plenty of things that get in the way of therapy. Some examples are:

- Being late on a regular basis
- Not showing up for sessions
- Not doing the homework
- Not practicing the skills

- Failing to complete the diary cards
- Using alcohol and drug
- Attending sessions under the influence
- Lying or omitting important information
- Derailing the therapy
- Failing to pay fees
- Generating crises
- Harming themselves
- Making suicide attempts
- Not talking about what's important until the end of the session
- Engaging in problematic behavior in and out of the session

A variety of strategies can be utilized to deal with these behaviors. Some of them are: acknowledge it, talk about it, use the informed consent effectively, leverage the therapeutic relationship, tap into the client's strengths, and use behavioral contracting, as well as applying natural and logical consequences when appropriate.

Clinicians, and the treatment system, sometimes engage in therapy interference as well. Some examples include:

- Not being physically or emotionally present in the session
- Answering the phone or checking e-mail during the session
- Starting late or running over regularly
- Falling asleep during the session
- Doing more talking than listening
- Getting hooked by crises
- Being judgmental with the client
- Allowing unchecked countertransference
- Being out of balance in the therapeutic relationship
- Failing to maintain optimal self-care
- Engaging in unhealthy co-dependency
- Breaching confidentiality
- Failing to maintain effective boundaries
- Getting personal needs met by the client
- Engaging in inappropriate relationships

Clinicians can minimize these therapy-interfering behaviors by staying in balance in the relationship, practicing self-care, and utilizing supervision, consultation, and peer support. Using their own DBT skills in their professional role is also helpful. Reducing or eliminating clinician-driven therapy interference can be facilitated by having less of the anti-DBT tactics while increasing effective clinician characteristics and skills on the following pages.

Review the following lists. Clinicians and treatment teams should consider how they can utilize fewer of the anti-DBT tactics and more of the effective clinician characteristics and skills.

ANTI-DBT TACTICS	EFFECTIVE CLINICIAN CHARACTERISTICS AND SKILLS
1. Call or think of the client as a manipulator	1. Hold a balance of the client's strengths and areas for growth
2. Communicate to the client how to feel, act, think	2. Have thorough knowledge of skills
3. Tell the client that other people should be different	3. Develop stories and metaphors to facilitate skill training
4. Tell the client what his are feelings	4. Plan for resistance to using skills or staying the course with the DBT process
5. Accuse the client of playing games or of not trying	5. Role-play skills in session
6. Accuse the client of splitting, either directly or to other staff	6. Assign skills practice as homework
7. Criticize the client's feelings	7. Review homework assignments
8. Encourage the client to mask emotions, or reinforce attempts to escape or avoid emotions	8. Provide coaching and encouragement for effective skills implementation
9. Stress the irrationality or distorted basis of his feelings	9. Be comfortable with ambiguity
10. Use the clinician's interpretations to attack, blame, or punish the client	10. Empower clients
11. Respond to painful feelings as something to get rid of	11. Avoid viewing the client or talking about the client in negative terms
12. Tell the client that problems are all in the mind	12. Accept client "as is" while encouraging change
13. Oversimplify the client's problems, implying that all will be well	13. Be centered and firm, while being flexible when appropriate
14. Push a particular set of values or philosophy of reality and truth	14. Establish clear limits of acceptable behavior
15. Present a rigid view of events	15. Adopt a non-defensive attitude

ANTI-DBT TACTICS	EFFECTIVE CLINICIAN CHARACTERISTICS AND SKILLS
16. Insist on one version of reality	16. Help clients analyze factors that inhibit or interfere with effort and motivation
17. Be judgmental of the client's choice of goals or commitments	17. Manage therapeutic transitions effectively
18. Impose the clinician's goals on the client	18. Assist clients in managing change and things that are out of their control
19. Be rigid about goals or procedures to reach goals	19. Practice good self-care
20. Be punitive	20. Effectively manage countertransference
21. Require behaviors beyond the client's capabilities	21. Utilize supervision, consultation and therapy when needed
22. Operate in a non-collaborative manner	22. Practice DBT skills yourself
23. When problem solving, ignore what the client can do in the situation	23. Foster dialectical thinking while compassionately confronting non-dialectical thinking
24. Overload the client with information	24. Suggest alternatives ways of thinking and interpreting reality
25. Get into a power struggle with the client	25. Facilitate and maintain dialectics in the therapeutic relationship

1. How can clinicians avoid anti-DBT tactics and achieve more effective clinician characteristics and skills?

   _____

   _____

   _____

2. How can colleagues and peers avoid anti-DBT tactics and achieve more effective clinician characteristics and skills?

   _____

   _____

   _____

3. How can the treatment team avoid anti-DBT tactics and achieve more effective clinician characteristics and skills?

   _____

   _____

   _____

4. How can agencies or organizations avoid anti-DBT tactics and achieve more effective clinician characteristics and skills?

   _____

   _____

   _____

TO BUILD A LIFE WORTH LIVING

Another dialectic of DBT is that while it is designed for severe pathology, it is also a strength-based model because the ultimate goal is to build a life worth living. The theory is that if clients build a life worth living they will be less inclined to engage in problematic, destructive behaviors.

Another way to think about having a life worth living is that a life worth living is a life in recovery. Recovery may include being abstinent from alcohol and drugs for clients who have an addiction but recovery is not limited to substance addictions only. Recovery has been expanded beyond the traditional 12-step perspective. Recovery is about clients being at the highest level of functioning, having optimal lifestyle and being the most well adjusted they can be even with mental health difficulties and other problems. The recovery paradigm is being adopted by the National Alliance of Mentally Ill (NAMI), the National Institute of Mental Health (NIMH), the Substance Abuse and Mental Health Services Administration (SAMHSA), state human services offices, county mental health departments, human services graduate programs, acute care systems, treatment programs, and private practice clinicians. A life in recovery is about clients living beyond their diagnoses and problems. A life in recovery is a holistic, comprehensive wellness perspective. It is about empowerment. It is about the client being the best he can be, at his highest level of functioning, or developing an optimal lifestyle. It is about each client and family reaching full potential.

While many of these ideas apply to clients with BPD, they also apply to other diagnostic categories of clients seeking therapy or treatment. Whether clients qualify for BPD diagnoses or just have impairments in their lives, DBT may provide the relief they seek and the opportunity to have the types of lives they would like to have. DBT was designed for a clinical population with severe problems and significant skills deficits but it is also helpful with a more moderate population such as clients with Axis I disorders, GAF scores above 65, and V code categories. DBT can help nearly any client to increase his level of functioning, improve communication, and increase life satisfaction.

DBT is a complex theory that combines many different components. At its core, DBT is a solid Cognitive Behavioral Therapy (CBT). As much as 60% of DBT is made up of CBT philosophies and interventions. Another significant part of DBT is the idea of balancing dialectics, which accounts for approximately 20% of the model. The last component of DBT, mindfulness, makes up the final 20% of the model. Mindfulness as a therapeutic process is gaining widespread acclaim. It has been integrated into the third wave of CBT, which includes Mindfulness-Based Stress Reduction, Mindfulness-Based Cognitive Therapy, and Acceptance and Commitment Therapy. This third wave focuses on secondary change, when clients make significant changes in their lives to support their new skills and perspectives. They adjust their thoughts, feelings, behaviors, and relationships in response to their newfound effectiveness, as well as focus on ways to sustain their new functioning.

THE SKILLS MODULES

MINDFULNESS

Being in the here and now is part of mindfulness. A focus on the here and now can be found in many models, such as Gestalt Therapy, as well as other therapeutic modalities, Western religions, and Eastern spiritual practices. Mindfulness is also about maintaining awareness—awareness of the internal experiences of sensations, energy levels, thoughts, emotions, and impulses as well as awareness of the external experiences in terms of what's going on in the environment and with interactions. Mindfulness is about staying present in the moment on both the inside and the outside to minimize interpretations, assumptions, abstractions, and judgments. When clients spend a considerable amount of energy thinking about what is going on, they may become hypervigilant and reactive to what they think is going on, which may be different from what is actually happening. Mindfulness is about getting out of thinking and into actual experiences. By being grounded in the here and now, clients are able to respond to what is going on, on both the inside and the outside. They are empowered to act in their own best interests.

Mindfulness in DBT is also about balance—balancing emotions, thoughts, behaviors, and relationships in the here and now as well as balancing the present with the past and the future. Some clients spend a considerable amount of time in the past. They may ruminate, analyze, and find themselves "less-than." The future, for other clients, is all-consuming. These clients catastrophize, worry about what will happen, and beat themselves up for not having other options. Then there are a third group of clients who spend a majority of their time in both the past and the future. For the clients that spend most of their time in the past or the future, there may be a strong sensation that life is passing them by. This may be an accurate perception since they spend a significant amount of time dwelling on the past or the future and not much time in the here and now.

Mindfulness emphasizes spending the majority of time in the present moment although it does allow for a focus on the past or the future. Being in the past or the future is done mindfully and with intention, and then the client returns to the here and now when they are done. Clients can reflect upon, learn from, and make sense of the past. Clients can also plan, prepare, and invest in the future. Staying connected to the past and the future can be productive when done in a mindful way rather than in ways that are distracting, intrusive, overwhelming, and distressing. Mindfulness is about voluntarily, intentionally paying attention to the current moment in a nonjudgmental fashion. It is voluntary in that clients are choosing to do it. It is intentional in that they are actively focusing their attention on the here and now.

With DBT's mindfulness skills, clients learn to be nonjudgmental. The nonjudgmental skill is about not assigning a value to yourself or others. The client is not good or bad. Clients often judge themselves as unlovable, damaged, evil, or imperfect. They may judge others as worthwhile, superior, and perfect while finding ways to judge themselves as less-than. They may hold themselves to higher standards than they hold others to. When their standards are unachievable for the average person it is a setup for failure.

This is a way for some clients to confirm their judgments. Being judgmental drives problematic, destructive behavior. If the client is unworthy or evil, shouldn't he be unhappy and in pain? This faulty logic justifies engaging in behavior that makes their lives worse and more painful. These clients can then judge their dysfunctional lives as confirmation that they are unlovable, damaged, and unworthy. This is circular thinking that begets a self-fulfilling prophecy.

Positive judgments may seem acceptable however, they are also problematic. Placing a value on oneself or others as good, deserving, or perfect is a slippery slope. It can easily lead to negative judgments. Positive judgments can feel inaccurate or false. Clients may judge themselves as impostors and frauds. Positive judgments can foster arrogance and looking down on others.

Being nonjudgmental is an ideal to strive for. It is not a concrete achievement that can be accomplished one day and then it is done for the foreseeable future. It is something to be worked on every day. There are days that clients will be more effective with being nonjudgmental and other days they will be less so. They will still judge sometimes, in small and big ways. An important point is to not be judgmental with themselves when they identify that they are being judgmental. This would be like rubbing salt in the wound—making the situation worse than it needs to be. It would double their judgments, because they would find themselves judging and then judge themselves for judging. An alternative is to identify the judgments, be compassionate toward themselves and recommit to being as nonjudgmental as possible.

Clients can learn to be nonjudgmental with themselves and others however they can't stop other people from judging them. Clients will benefit from developing the ability to let others' judgments roll off them, rather than letting them "stick" and take hold in their self-images. It will also be effective if clients can avoid judging others who are judging them.

Individuals are not good or bad, though their behavior may be good, bad, useful, problematic, healthy, destructive, inappropriate, or wrong. Behavior can be judged, but it doesn't mean anything about the value of the individual. Behavior that is problematic, inappropriate, or wrong typically has natural and logical consequences. Natural and logical consequences help to negatively reinforce the problematic, inappropriate, or wrong behavior. The client should understand that the expectation is to move away from this behavior towards life-enhancing behaviors.

It is crucial to figure out what purpose the problematic, destructive behavior serves. When the purpose is to confirm their judgments, DBT teaches clients to be nonjudgmental with themselves and others. Other needs are modulating pain, providing intensity, feeling alive, and getting support from others. DBT helps the client learn to replace his problematic, self-destructive behaviors with DBT skills that will meet these needs without the costs or damages caused by current strategies. The skills contained in the Mindfulness, Distress Tolerance, Emotional

Regulation, Interpersonal Effectiveness, and Middle Path categories can provide the tools necessary to be successful in being nonjudgmental.

DISTRESS TOLERANCE

In the traditional DBT model the distress tolerance module is third because it is a subgroup of skills under the emotional regulation umbrella. But teaching these skills sooner rather than later meets the clients where they are and provides them the opportunity for relief. Crises and distress are the causes that typically bring individuals and families into therapy: clients and their families want assistance as well as solutions to the problems they are experiencing. The skills contained in this module provide them with tools to cope, manage, distract, and tolerate crises, stress, and drama.

Distress tolerance is about frustration tolerance. Frustration tolerance is a developmental milestone typically experienced in adolescence. Adult clients who have experienced disrupted development, abuse, or trauma may also be attempting to successfully complete this milestone. Frustration tolerance means being able to hold frustration and stress without engaging in negative, problematic, or destructive behaviors. Some frustrations can be tolerated while other frustrations can be modulated.

Part of frustration tolerance is moving away from willfulness. Willfulness is a mindset that clients may have: they want it their way just because they do. Willfulness is also about the feelings and behaviors that go along with the mindset of "my way or the highway." Sometimes clients want what they want without any solid reasoning behind their desire. Willfulness is fleeting and the client getting what he wants doesn't last long enough so then the client has to want something else. Willfulness usually comes with a cost to energy level, relationships, and quality of life. Willfulness also tells clients that when they don't get what they want they are failures.

By comparison, distress tolerance encourages clients to be willing. Willingness teaches that sometimes the client gets it his way, sometimes others get it their way, and whenever possible both getting their way is optimal. Willingness takes the ability to tolerate hearing "no" or being disappointed. Sometimes the client not getting what he wants is the most useful lesson and can lead to an unexpected outcome. Willingness is about collaboration. It is about trusting the process and letting go of control. It is about not sweating the small stuff. It is energy-generating, fosters relationships, and increases quality of life.

EMOTIONAL REGULATION

In this module clients learn about their emotions, achieve a deeper understanding of their emotional life, and develop more resiliency when dealing with emotions. Emotions are part of life. Sometimes clients believe that they shouldn't have any emotions, or that they should only have positive emotions. When they have negative emotions such anger, sadness, or loneliness they may feel that they have to get rid of them. They judge themselves by the emotions they experience.

Two major components of this module are assisting clients to learn impulse control and to delay gratification. Part of the process is having clients realize that they can feel an impulse or strong emotion but not act on it. They can learn to tolerate the impulse or emotion, which would be **Riding the Wave**. By **Riding the Wave**, they are harnessing the energy, impulse, or emotion, staying mindfully present with it, and being patient until it shifts into the next impulse or emotion in the same way waves rise and fall.

In addition to **Riding the Wave**, clients can choose to use a DBT skill to deal with the impulse. Or they can choose to act on the impulse or emotion in a less harmful way. Finally, they can choose to act on the impulse at full strength. In this last option, they are actively choosing to engage with it instead of feeling as if it is happening on autopilot or as if they are merely reacting to it.

INTERPERSONAL EFFECTIVENESS

In this module clients learn how to have functional relationships. According to DBT there are three types of interpersonal effectiveness: Objective, Relationship, and Self-Respect (Linehan 1993a; Linehan 1993b).

Objective effectiveness is about clients getting what they want in relationships, meeting a need, or accomplishing an objective. Clients learn how to ask for help and how to tolerate not always getting what they want. Relationship effectiveness is about building healthy, respectful, and responsive relationships. Self-respect effectiveness is about being able to identify one's needs and get them met. Relationship and self-respect effectiveness form a dialectic: balancing self and others, giving and getting. They are about healthy co-dependence. The skills in this module help clients balance their needs with the needs of others. This empowers them to communicate in clear and respectful ways, as well as helps them to deal with difficult or challenging people with whom they interact.

THE MIDDLE PATH

This module that is commonly used with teenagers and families (Miller, 2006). It doesn't contain specific skills but instead pulls any and all skills from other modules and teaches them for use in a family system. It is also about educating teenagers and families about having balance in their relationships. It assists families in achieving balance, particularly with boundaries and discipline. This module also teaches families how to hold dialectics and avoid power struggles about dichotomies. An example would be working with families to help them avoid getting into "always/never" arguments. Another area for balance in families is acceptance and change. Each member in the family learns to accept himself and others while also engaging in changed behaviors that support individual and family goals. For definitions of the skills mentioned below, see Chapter 3. Additional dialectics are:

- Excessive leniency vs. Authoritarian control
- Normalizing pathological behaviors vs. Pathologizing normative behaviors
- Forcing autonomy vs. Fostering dependence

The excessive leniency vs. authoritarian control can be broken down into two more concrete subgroups of dialectics. The first one is about increasing authoritative discipline while decreasing excessive leniency. This can be accomplished through:

- Mindfulness: ***Wise Mind***
- Distress Tolerance: ***ACCEPTS***
- Emotional Regulation: ***Build Positive Emotions***
- Interpersonal Effectiveness: ***Broken Records***

The second subgroup of dialectics in this category is when parents facilitate self-determination in the adolescents while decreasing authoritarian control in parenting. This can be accomplished by:

- Mindfulness: ***Body Scan***
- Distress Tolerance: ***Radical Acceptance***
- Emotional Regulation: ***MEDDSS***
- Interpersonal Effectiveness: ***Relationship Assumptions***

The second major category of dialectics is normalizing pathological behaviors vs. pathologizing normative behaviors. Within this dialectic there are also two more concrete subgroups of dialectics. The first one is increasing recognition of normative behaviors while decreasing pathologizing of normative behaviors. This can be accomplished by:

- Mindfulness: ***One-Mindfully***
- Distress Tolerance: ***IMPROVES***
- Emotional Regulation: ***EMOTIONS***
- Interpersonal Effectiveness: ***Relationship Mindfulness***

The next subgroup of dialectics is increasing identification of problem behaviors while decreasing normalization of problem behaviors. This can be accomplished by:

- Mindfulness: ***Be Mindful***
- Distress Tolerance: ***Pros & Cons***
- Emotional Regulation: ***TRUST***
- Interpersonal Effectiveness: ***Difficult People***

The final dialectic for families is forcing autonomy vs. fostering dependence. The first subgroup of dialectics within this category is increasing individuation while decreasing excessive dependence. This can be accomplished by:

- Mindfulness: ***Turtling***
- Distress Tolerance: ***Moment to Pause***
- Emotional Regulation: ***Opposite to Emotions***
- Interpersonal Effectiveness: ***FAST***

The second subgroup of dialectics here is increasing effective reliance on others while decreasing excessive autonomy. This can be accomplished by:

- Mindfulness: **Observe/Describe**
- Distress Tolerance: **Feeling not Acting**
- Emotional Regulation: **Ride the Wave**
- Interpersonal Effectiveness: **GIVE**

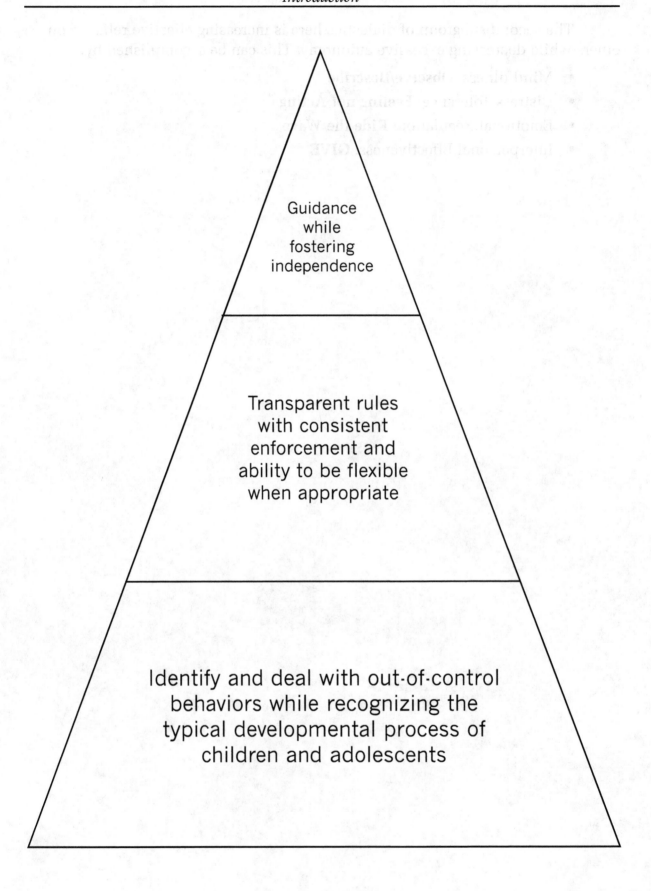

Guidance while fostering independence

Transparent rules with consistent enforcement and ability to be flexible when appropriate

Identify and deal with out-of-control behaviors while recognizing the typical developmental process of children and adolescents

META SKILLS

The meta-skills are a selection of skills that encapsulate the philosophy and essential strategies of DBT (Moonshine, 2007). These are skills that draw on each of the four content areas to provide comprehensive solutions for clients. These may be the most important of all of the DBT skills as they work together to empower clients to build a life worth living. The meta-skills are:

- *MEDDSS*
- *Effectively*
- *Wise Mind*
- *IPE—GIVE-FAST—DEAR WOMAN*
- *Nonjudgmental*
- *Radical Acceptance*

Together these skills create a whole way of living which is more than just the sum of its parts. It is a holistic strategy for living in the moment, effectively managing distress, having flexibility in emotional expression, and applying skills to engage in functional relationships.

META-SKILLS

Skills	Description					
MEDDSS	Mastery	Exercise	Diet	Drugs	Sleep	Spirituality

Effectively	• Working to be as effective as we can be in our lives. • Identifying what is more effective and avoiding less effective strategies and behaviors in our lives. • Avoiding judgmental words such as better, worse, good, or bad.
Wise Mind	• Balancing Rational Mind and Emotional Mind to create Wise Mind. • We are able to be most mindful and effective when we can have both Rational and Emotional Mind present in our experience. Be sure not to judge Rational Mind as good and Emotional Mind as bad. Neither is good or bad, just part of our experience in life. • By being in Wise Mind, we are in balance and have all our senses, ways of knowing, and skills at our disposal to manage our lives effectively and to act in our best interests.

Interpersonal Effectiveness (IPE)	**GIVE**	Gentle	Interested	Validate	Easy Manner	
	FAST	Fair to Self	Apologize Less	Stick to Values	Truthful with Self	
	DEAR WOMAN or MAN	Describe	Encourage	Ask	Reinforce	
		Willingness	Observe	Mindful	Appear Confident	Negotiate

Non-Judgmental	• Suspending evaluations about self and others. • Judging behavior as right or wrong, good or bad, but not judging the person engaging in the behavior. Behavior can generate natural and logical consequences but we don't label the person engaging in the behavior. • Describing things concretely, in non-judgmental terms. • Liking or disliking things while not judging ourselves or others. • Holding values that are beliefs or ethics, not judgments.
Radical Acceptance	• The Serenity Prayer • We do not have the ability to control others' thoughts, feelings, and actions. • We may have limited control over what happens around us and what others do. • We can effectively focus our attention and energy on what we can control and change: ourselves.

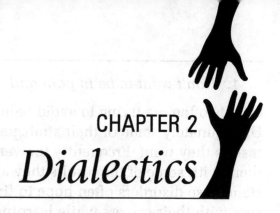

CHAPTER 2
Dialectics

Dialectics are about holding in balance things that seem to be contradictory, mismatched, in direct competition with each other, or in conflict. Ironies and paradoxes are dialectics. Dialectics are ways that reality is black, white, and many shades of gray. There are times when there is more than one right answer and other times when there is no single right answer. Life is full of inconsistencies and contradictions. However, both clients and clinicians can learn to think and act dialectically. In other words, they can actively work toward balance in a variety of ways. Balance is often about moving away from the extreme ends of the dialectic toward the middle. It can be about blending a little bit of both ends of the spectrum. One way to think about this is a synthesis of both sides of the dialectic. For each of the client's dialectics discussed there are suggested skills. See Chapter 3 for explanation of all skills.

CLIENT DIALECTICS

1. Don't want to be in pain and don't want to change

2. Believe that reality is out of their control, while continuing to engage in controlling behavior

3. Want their lives to be better while still want to engage in problematic self-destructive behavior

4. Want life to be easy and spend a lot of energy making it harder than it needs to be

5. Demand respect while being disrespectful to others (and/or self!)

6. Want to be treated like an adult while behaving in immature ways

7. Focus on self-focusing and focus on others

8. Want help and reject support

9. Want spontaneity while life is full of obligations

10. Balance reactivity and responsivity

1. *Don't want to be in pain and don't want to change.*

Clients often are trying to avoid being in pain, or to have less chaos in their lives. Unfortunately some of their strategies are less than effective and don't produce the results they want. Frequently the very thing they don't want to do will provide them with some of the results they are looking for. For example, clients with substance use disorders often hope to find a way to have better relationships and success with their careers while learning to control or moderate their use rather than giving it up. While some clients can learn to use moderately, many cannot. For clients with out-of-control addictions, with their bio-psycho-social etiology, abstinence is recommended. These clients will not be able to achieve relationship or career success without abstinence. The more they try to control their use, the more control it has over them and perhaps the further away from their goals they find themselves; they will come closer to their goals only when they abstain completely. That said, with initial abstinence things often get worse before they get better because the client often has to deal with the wreckage of his addiction.

Another example might be teenagers who experience interpersonal drama. Teenagers have a sense of loyalty and want to trust their friends and rely on their relationships. Given this goal, it is curious that these same teenagers engage in gossip, indirect communication, and being judgmental with one another. The more they engage in these behaviors the more interpersonal drama they will have along with a decreased ability to rely on their relationships.

Developmentally, teenagers and young adults are focused on group membership. Their psychological development defines their identities which in turn is defined by who their friends are (and who they aren't), while physical development is characterized by growth hormones. This may lead to emotional reactivity and dysregulation. Clients may engage in self-destructive behavior such as cutting, burning themselves, banging their heads, getting in physical fights, raging out of control, driving aggressively, excessive use of alcohol and drugs, out-of-control spending, gambling, bingeing/purging, engaging in risky sexual behavior, or other behaviors. These clients may have a hard time tolerating psychological, emotional, and/or physical pain. Their self-destructive behaviors may be coping strategies to manage, distract, or deny some pain by creating other pain. For these clients clinicians recommend stopping the behaviors and replacing them with more functional coping strategies that can often include one or more DBT skills.

In many cases, clients don't want to change their behavior or they are unconvinced that there might be something more effective for coping with, managing, reducing, or eliminating their pain. Their self-destructive behaviors have been a survival strategy for managing their difficult or out-of-control life circumstances. These behaviors have been meeting a need despite costs such as physical harm, disappointing others, and diminished capacity to meet major life goals.

Balancing the dialectic of wanting less pain while avoiding change can occur when clients learn how to tolerate, cope with, and manage pain while engaging in change strategies. Ultimately this may lead to clients managing their lives more effectively, increasing their goal-directed behavior, and overall level of functioning.

- <u>Mindfulness</u>: Staying in the present moment.
  <u>Suggested Skill</u>: ***Observe and Describe***

- <u>Distress Tolerance</u>: Building frustration tolerance in order to tolerate the pain. Becoming empowered to do things differently even when it is difficult or challenging.
  <u>Suggested Skill</u>: ***Keeping It In Perspective***

- <u>Emotional Regulation</u>: Developing the ability to stay present with the emotions without engaging in problematic actions.
  <u>Suggested Skill</u>: ***ABC***

- <u>Interpersonal Effectiveness</u>: Staying connected to others even when in pain or stressed out.
  <u>Suggested Skill</u>: ***Broken Records***

2. *Believe that reality is out of their control while engaging in controlling behavior.*

Often clients experience their lives as being out of control. These individuals view life as happening to them. They are passive and perhaps even victims of whatever happens to them while at the same time they engage in considerable controlling behavior. Controlling behavior can manifest in wanting things to be a certain way or beliefs that others should think the same way. Other controlling behaviors can include, but aren't limited to: listening in on others' conversations, watching others, reading others' papers, over interpreting cues in the environment, enlisting allies to support interpretations, and investing a lot of energy in getting things their way.

An example might be the client who comes in on a regular basis complaining that bad things keep happening to him but he doesn't acknowledge that continuing to hang out with certain people will only lead to being taken advantage of. Other clients, who believe that people are out to get them, sometimes try to protect themselves by engaging in intimidating behaviors that may provoke others to attack them emotionally, interpersonally, or perhaps even physically.

Clients can learn to control what they do have control over: themselves. Clients can learn to manage their own thoughts, emotions, impulses, and behaviors. They can learn to influence others and their environments while investing most of their energy into their own thinking, feelings, impulses, and actions. Letting go of their attempts to control others and the environment can empower clients to take better care of themselves by redirecting their energy away from things they are powerless over and toward what the only thing they do have power over: themselves.

Balancing the dialectic of being more in control without being controlling can be accomplished by clients' accepting the fact that they have control over themselves and influence on others and the environment while also accepting the fact that they can't control others or the environment. This balance empowers clients to focus their time, energy, and attention on managing their own lives effectively.

- Mindfulness: Being present with yourself, inside and outside, so you can focus your energy on effectively managing your life.
  Suggested Skill: ***One Mindfully***

- Distress Tolerance: Learning to let go and move away from areas where you don't have influence. Being able to tolerate not getting it your way all the time. Being curious about and open to unexpected positives coming from not getting it your way.
  Suggested Skill: ***Willingness***

- Emotional Regulation: Learning to cope with and manage emotions and impulses in order to build a life worth living.
  Suggested Skill: ***Feeling Not Acting***

- Interpersonal Effectiveness: Investing in relationships even when you realize that you cannot control how other people think, feel, or behave.
  Suggested Skill: ***4 Horsemen***

3. *Want their lives to be better while still engaging in problematic self-destructive behaviors.*

Many clients come to treatment asking for help to have fewer problems and more life satisfaction. They may present with ideas they want to work on. They may have specific goals on which they want to make progress. They may have a vision for their future.

At the same time, many of these clients are unwilling to give up their problematic behavior. This behavior has helped them to manage their chaotic, out-of-control lives. In extreme cases, clients have been using the problematic behavior as a survival strategy to manage their pain, distress, and dangerous environments. In less severe cases, clients engaging in problematic behavior might minimize its damage and overestimate its benefits.

What are some examples of this dialectic? Clients who want to have better relationships with family members but rage out of control. Clients who actively engage in strategies to have fewer crises while cutting or burning themselves or making suicide attempts. Teenagers and young adults might work hard at school to plan a future while withdrawing from relationships and failing to engage in effective self-care behaviors.

Balancing the dialectic of wanting life to be better while struggling to reduce or eliminate problematic behavior can occur by exploring the pros and cons of behavior, replacing extreme behavior with more effective behavior, and appreciating the concerns others may have about their behavior.

- Mindfulness: Being in the here and now empowers you to deal with environmental and interpersonal realities.
  Suggested Skill: ***Moment to Pause***

- Distress Tolerance: Utilizing the active strategies in this module provides you with many opportunities to be more effective even in the midst of stress, drama, and crisis.
  Suggested Skill: ***Exploring Pros and Cons***

- Emotional Regulation: Being mindfully present with the impulse to engage in problematic behavior without acting on it. You can choose to tolerate the impulse or use skills to modulate it.
  Suggested Skill: ***Lemonade***

- Interpersonal Effectiveness: You can use your skills to balance objective, relationship, and self-respect effectiveness in primary, intimate, and casual relationships.
  Suggested Skill: ***Relationship Mindfulness***

4. *Want life to be easy and spend a lot of energy making it harder than it needs to be.*

Individuals holding this dialectic are hoping that life will be easier, less stressful and without problems. They would like to have less stress at work, school, home, in relationships, and perhaps even financially, but these same individuals make choices and behave in ways that make their lives harder than they need to be. Some examples are clients who engage in argumentative or combative behavior, clients who behave inappropriately at work or school, or clients who spend beyond their means.

Another example is a client who says she is committed to effectively managing stress but who over-commits and doesn't leave sufficient time for adequate self-care. Or a client who decides that having less interpersonal drama in his life will be useful, but continues to gossip and talk negatively about co-workers or classmates. A third example would be a client whose judgment of himself as being damaged fuels his self-destructive behavior, but who talks about how being non-judgmental of others has significantly improved relationships with family and friends.

Balancing the dialectic of wanting life to be easy and engaging in behavior that makes things harder can be accomplished by clients remembering that while they're doing the best they can, they can try harder, increase their skills, and be more effective.

- Mindfulness: Staying out of the failures of the past and future empowers you to be more effective in the here and now. This is also facilitated by balancing immediate, short-term, and long-term perspectives.
  Suggested Skill: ***Be Mindful***

- Distress Tolerance: By being able to tolerate distress and frustration, you can suspend the behaviors that make things worse.
  Suggested Skill: ***SPECIFIC PATHS***

- Emotional Regulation: These skills, combined with distress tolerance, teach you that you have alternatives to your patterns of ineffective behavior.
  Suggested Skill: ***EMOTIONS***

- Interpersonal Effectiveness: These skills teach you how to have healthy relationships.
  Suggested Skill: ***Relationship Thinking***

5. *Demand respect while being disrespectful.*

Everyone has a desire to be respected. For some clients this is extremely important. These individuals scrutinize the way others interact with them: the words spoken, tone of voice, and nonverbal behaviors. All of this is evaluated as being respectful or disrespectful. When a client determines that he is being treated disrespectfully he may react toward others or himself in verbally or physically ways.

Sometimes these same individuals behave in ways that are disrespectful to others. This can include the specific words used, tones of voice, body posture, gestures, and eye contact among others. These behaviors can produce reactions from others that are then interpreted as disrespectful and even provocative. This will encourage the client to engage in more of the same type of behavior. In extreme cases it becomes an escalating situation that may end in threats, destruction of property, or violence toward others.

An example would be a teenager who interprets another teen's tone of voice and eye contact as disrespectful and starts a physical altercation. Another client may feel disrespected at work and retaliate by choosing not to complete an assignment that results in team members being frustrated, less collaborative, and perhaps actively trying to discredit the client. Yet another client might accuse his spouse of being disrespectful while using negative, offensive, and disrespectful language himself.

Clients can balance the dialectic of expecting respect and tolerating disrespect while behaving respectfully by paying attention to their own word choices, tones of voice, gestures, eye contact, and behavior while reducing or eliminating assumptions or interpretations of others' intentions or behaviors.

- Mindfulness: Staying grounded in the here and now internally, in their environment, and in your interactions to avoid making interpretations or assumptions.
  Suggested Skill: ***Effectively***

- Distress Tolerance: Learning to tolerate situations where disrespect has occurred.
  Suggested Skill: ***IMPROVE***

- Emotional Regulation: Empowers you to be more effective by moving away from your own disrespectful behavior and ignoring the disrespectful behavior of others.
  Suggested Skill: ***TRUST***

- Interpersonal Effectiveness: Staying connected in relationships even if there has been disrespect on either side of the fence.
  Suggested Skill: ***Difficult People***

6. *Want to be treated like an adult while behaving in immature ways.*

While this may most often apply to teenagers, it can also apply to kids and even adults at times. In this situation clients want to be treated like adults and to be independent, make their own decisions, and manage their own behavior. These same clients may have difficulty making decisions and be unable to regulate their impulses or modulate their emotions.

Some examples include teenagers who don't want their parents checking their online behavior while the teenagers are talking online to people they don't know and who might prove to be unsafe; a young adult who stays out late in dangerous parts of town but tells everyone that he is OK and can take of himself; or a kid who wants to be helpful to his parents and to be seen as a big kid but who bullies his younger siblings.

Balancing the dialectic of wanting to be treated like an adult but acting immaturely sometimes can be achieved by learning to be assertive, engaging in appropriate behavior, building confidence in oneself, and earning confidence from others over time. The ability to not have all the answers and to ask for help are important parts of being an adult. And being able to have fun and not grow up too fast is a major component of the process as well.

- Mindfulness: Staying in the moment so that you don't get ahead of yourself.
  Suggested Skill: ***Participate***

- Distress Tolerance: Effectively managing frustration tolerance and bouncing back from stressful situations are essential competencies for adulthood.
  Suggested Skill: ***Self-Soothe First-Aid Kit***

- Emotional Regulation: The ability to tolerate and cope with strong emotions and impulses are also requisite competencies for adulthood.
  Suggested Skill: ***Love Dandelions***

- Interpersonal Effectiveness: Adulthood is characterized by relationships that ebb, flow, sometimes end, and endure.
  Suggested Skill: ***Repairs***

7. *Focus on self and focus on others.*

Some clients spend most of their time and energy focusing on themselves while other clients spend enormous amounts of time and energy focusing on others. Both of these perspectives are inherently out of balance. Other-focusing behavior may be observed when clients spend all their time taking care of partners or family members but don't invest enough time in self-care, downtime, or having fun. They put their own needs on the back burner, doing favors and dropping everything to help out someone else. Another client may always expect others to help him but does little for others. Self-focusing clients may obsess about a particular component of their own lives such as attractiveness, their career, or accumulating money.

It is entirely possible for clients to be able to balance their focus between themselves and others as well as to balance giving and receiving. This might be thought of as healthy co-dependence and it can be achieved by knowing oneself, being able to set limits, and not allowing guilt feelings to drive behavior into overdoing for others.

- Mindfulness: Being in the here and now can empower you to stay grounded in your strategies to balance your focus between yourself and others.
  Suggested Skill: ***Nonjudgmental***

- Distress Tolerance: You can learn to manage your own needs and desires along with others' requests and demands.
  Suggested Skill: ***Half Smile***

- Emotional Regulation: Your ability to balance self and others or giving and receiving can require significant competency with emotional regulation.
  Suggested Skill: ***MEDDSS***

- Interpersonal Effectiveness: This domain provides critical skills to achieve balance by investing in self and investing in relationships with others.
  Suggested Skill: ***GIVE/FAST***

8. *Want help and reject support.*

Here clients communicate directly or indirectly that they need help yet they often reject the assistance that people offer. It may appear that the client is generating a crisis and that any help offered by others would be insufficient in the client's mind. Clients feel invalidated because others don't understand the details of their lives. They may interpret others' inability to help them as confirming some negative judgment about themselves or a belief that they deserve to be miserable and in pain.

A depressed client's family members may suggest getting out of bed, being active, and taking antidepressants, while in fact the client feels incapable of doing even one of these things let alone all three. Or the client and family members may collude in the perceived hopelessness of the situation. Another client, struggling with addiction, may want to stop, to not be in so much pain, and not disappoint his family. Yet he finds reasons to pass up community supports such as 12-step groups, drops out of a treatment program, and begins hanging out with others who get high. This client may be very aware that this behavior puts his recovery at risk, but that doesn't resonate with him and he believes he has no other choice but to continue to use.

Balancing the dialectic of wanting help and having a difficulty accepting it can be achieved by learning to sometimes accept help even if it doesn't seem like it would be helpful. Another component of this process may be learning to actively deal with a problem even when it doesn't completely resolve the issue. There also may be times when tolerating a painful situation is warranted; on these occasions it is important to not communicate to others that help is requested since the client has no intention of acting on it just yet.

- Mindfulness: The present moment provides an opportunity to decide what is really wanted and to engage in the behavior, whether it is getting help to change or learning to be OK with the way things are without changing.
  Suggested Skill: ***Turtling***

- Distress Tolerance: Being able to tolerate the fact that things don't always get better and that sometimes others want to help even when they aren't really helpful.
  Suggested Skill: ***Self Soothe***

- Emotional Regulation: These skills help you stay grounded in your life even when things don't seem to improve or when there are no useful answers.
  Suggested Skill: ***Ride the Wave***

- Interpersonal Effectiveness: Here you learn how to effectively stay in relationships without rejecting others.
  Suggested Skill: ***DEAR WOMAN***

9. *Want spontaneity while life is full of obligations.*

Many clients have a long list of obligations that demand the majority of their time, energy, and attention. These same clients may want to have few or no obligations. They may crave spontaneity. Other clients have lots of spontaneity and live largely unstructured lives. These clients may experience life as ungrounded and with little meaning.

Both of these clients will benefit from having a little bit of what the other experiences. Balance occurs when clients are not at one extreme or the other. Here it is important to work with overburdened clients to reduce life obligations where possible. An important part of this process may be accepting the self, others, and the world around them as imperfect. Being able to say no and set appropriate limits will be useful with this dialectic. Clients at the other extreme may need help to be able to find meaning in structure and occasional hard work.

- Mindfulness: Being in the moment with both obligations and spontaneity takes intentional mindfulness.
  Suggested Skill: ***ONE MIND***

- Distress Tolerance: Managing the frustration and exhaustion of excessive obligations can be accomplished with these skills.
  Suggested Skill: ***ACCEPTS***

- Emotional Regulation: The ability to delay gratification learned from these skills will be useful with this dialectic.
  Suggested Skill: ***EMOTIONS***

- Interpersonal Effectiveness: Empowers you to be present in your relationships while balancing demands.
  Suggested Skill: ***Ignore***

10. *Balance reactivity and responsivity.*

Some clients live their lives in a reactive manner. They are often having crises—things just aren't going their way. They have learned to be hypervigilant so that they can figure out what is going on and then react as quickly as possible. In these situations clients will benefit from getting out of this reactive mindset. The ability to be responsive to life more often, rather than reactive, increases a client's effectiveness in a variety of domains.

Clients can balance the dialectic of managing reactivity while still being responsive by staying focused on what is going on internally, around them, and in interactions with others while suspending the need to make assumptions, interpretations, reactions, and judgments.

- Mindfulness: Staying in the moment helps you to remain grounded in actual experience on the inside and in what is going on around you, rather than in what you imagine is going on.
  Suggested Skill: ***Wise Mind***

- Distress Tolerance: Learning to effectively deal with difficulty and painful situations is accomplished by these skills.
  Suggested Skill: ***Crisis Survival Network***

- Emotional Regulation: The impulse control fostered through these skills reduces reactivity.
  Suggested Skill: ***Opposite to Emotions***

- Interpersonal Effectiveness: You can use these skills to establish self-respect and relationship effectiveness.
  Suggested Skill: ***Pay it Forward***

CLIENT DIALECTICS CONCLUSION

DBT is about balance. It empowers clients to see that reality is black and white as well as a lot of shades of gray. It is about helping clients to hold in balance things that are contrary, confusing, or in conflict, and yet are real or true for them. Balancing the dialectic happens intrapsychically and interpersonally. It also happens between the client and various environments. It is about the clients' being able to tolerate and manage the ambiguity of life. It is about accepting that they may have competing needs, such as being independent versus being taken care of, while achieving the optimal balance with each need. It is also about clients accepting that life is imperfect and taking control over what they have control over: their own energy level, thoughts, feelings, impulses, and behaviors.

CLINICIAN DIALECTICS

1. Using evidence-based practices while individualizing treatment.

2. Being culturally competent while using empirically validated practices.

3. Remaining relationship oriented while completing paperwork and insurance reviews.

4. Encouraging clients to engage in more effective self-care while maintaining sufficient self-care practices oneself.

5. Diagnosing and seeing deficits and having a strength-based perspective.

6. Wanting clients to change while not always being patient or positively reinforcing change.

7. Being critical of self while being compassionate toward others.

8. Being committed to professional endeavors and investing in personal life.

9. Being competent while having a lifelong commitment to learning.

10. Wanting to be good at DBT before being ready to invest the time and energy to do so.

1. *Using evidence-based practices while individualizing treatment.*

The mental health and addictions fields have long been committed to providing individualized treatment. This requires collaboration with clients to understand their lives, difficulties, hopes, and aspirations. Treatment planning and goal setting occur as the clinician and client get to know one another and agree upon steps in the treatment process. It is standard protocol that problems and goals be documented in the client's language and that there is documentation of other evidence of participation by the client and perhaps his family in the clinical record.

Recently there have been increasing mandates for clinicians, treatment centers, and human services to utilize evidence-based practices (EBPs). EBPs are empirically validated protocols that have been shown to produce positive outcomes. These mandates require that appropriate EBPs are used with the populations for which they are designed, and that they be applied, like a recipe, in the same way as they were researched. This process leaves little or no room for flexibility, creativity, or individualization.

Many EBPs have a fidelity tool that assesses how closely the treatment provided follows the research model. Often the fidelity tool includes direct observation of treatment services, interviews with clinical staff, program administrators, and clients as well as evidence in clinical documentation. Fidelity to the EBPs shows that they are being implemented consistently. Funding sources and government oversight agencies are increasingly expecting, and requiring, fidelity to the EBPs yet this would be the opposite of individualized treatment.

It is still early in the field's development to achieve balance with this dialectic. Some have written that it is essential to maintain the core components of EBP while being flexible enough to modify treatment when needed and build a strong therapeutic alliance. This dialectic is really about the shades of gray. The EBPs need to be recognizable and differentiated from other practices while also meeting the client where he is, and including his goals and desires as integral components of the treatment process. Clinicians and supervisors must maintain vigilance to ensure this balance is achieved and maintained.

2. *Being culturally competent while using empirically validated practices.*

Another dialectic with the commitment to use EBPs is cultural competency. Most EBPs have been researched using participants from the dominant culture which is primarily Caucasian, middle class, and heterosexual. Yet it is also important to understand and integrate a culturally diverse perspective into the interventions and services provided. A rubric for being responsive to diversity was developed by Pamela Hayes, Ph.D. In 2007, she published the ADDRESSING model.

- **A** = Age and generation
- **D** = Developmental Milestones
- **D** = Disability
- **R** = Religion and Spirituality
- **E** = Ethnicity and Race
- **S** = Socio-Economic Factors
- **S** = Sexual Orientation
- **I** = Indigenous Heritage
- **N** = Nationality
- **G** = Gender Identity and Role

(Hays, 2007)

This may not be a comprehensive rubric for diversity but it is considerably more inclusive than focusing on race and ethnicity alone. Diversity is a dynamic component of clients' and clinicians' lives. Many of the factors in the ADDRESSING model interact with one another and may also change over time. Each individual experiences his diversity components differently and interacts uniquely with other diverse individuals.

In many cases it would be considered inappropriate to provide treatment to minority-culture individuals with exclusively dominant-culture models. EBPs may not be appropriate for a diverse clientele that includes people of color, varying religious and spiritual or socio-economic backgrounds, sexual orientations, indigenous heritages, and ages or generations. All professional organizations hold clinicians accountable to treat every individual with care, respect, courtesy, and innovation. Again there is conflict between EBPs and culturally-responsive services.

3. *Remaining relationship oriented, while completing paperwork and insurance reviews.*

A strength of many clinicians is that they are relationship-oriented. They are able to build safe and intimate relationships with a variety of children, teenagers, adults, and older adults. While the research supports the use of EBPs, it also supports the importance of the therapeutic relationship. Some national figures suggest that it doesn't matter what EBP is used as long as there is a strong therapeutic alliance. In most cases change happens when both are present, which in itself is dialectical. It can easily be agreed upon by many clinicians that the relationship is a critical factor in the success of therapy or treatment.

Completing paperwork and insurance reviews may be a funding requirement and therefore a part of a clinician's job. In some situations this isn't the case, such as private practice clinicians who work only with self-pay clients or where public sector agencies are funded directly by foundations or government agencies. Even in these cases there may be laws, regulations, risk management protocols, and standards of care requiring that all treatment to be documented. Yet paperwork takes time away from clinical services. It may present a barrier to a strong therapeutic alliance because of the time and energy needed and the frustration sometimes caused by completing paperwork. And viewing paperwork as an unnecessary evil to be avoided will only facilitate the negative behavior of failing to adequately complete documentation.

Clinicians can balance this dialectic by maintaining the mindset that both the relationship and the paperwork are part of the clinical process. The first step is to view paperwork as clinical documentation. Clinicians will benefit from taking some time each day, when possible, to complete documentation and to make it a useful and accurate record of the treatment being provided. Individualized documentation may take more effort to create, yet in the end it will be more useful to the clinician, supervisor, insurance company, client, family members, and other members of the treatment team. Effectively managing time and reducing procrastination are two additional pieces to the puzzle that will help produce balance. It is recommended that individuals create documentation standards and forms that reduce redundancy and utilize technology to support a streamlined and efficient documentation process.

4. *Encouraging clients to engage in more effective self-care while clinicians maintain sufficient self-care practices.*

Establishing effective self-care regimens help clients manage stress and improve their lives. Self-care can include exercise, sufficient sleep, a healthy support system, and the ability to take care of oneself as well as activities of daily living like hygiene, medication compliance, and balanced nutrition. Some clients come into therapy or treatment with significant impairments or lack skills for effective self-care. Educating and assisting these clients to implement self-care on a daily basis is an essential part of the treatment process.

Some of the same clinicians who make self-care an important goal for their clients engage in ineffective, little, or no self-care themselves. Some clinicians believe that they must work as hard as possible, consistently giving more than 100% of themselves for their clients. This may be due to unchecked co-dependency issues or over-attachment to doing the work. A metaphor may be useful to illustrate the flaw in this behavior. Airplane passengers are instructed that if the oxygen masks drop down each passenger must put on his own mask first before helping others. Passengers who try to assist others first will likely pass out from lack of oxygen, ending their ability to help anyone.

The same is true for clinicians. If they are always helping others, they may burn out and leave the field. Additionally, taking too much care of others fosters dependence—the very opposite of empowering clients to take care of themselves.

Clinicians will make progress toward balance when they can "walk the talk" with the same dedication they encourage their clients to have. All of the same things that are helpful for clients are also helpful for clinicians: balanced nutrition, exercise, sleep, hygiene, healthy support systems, and the ability to take care of oneself. Because human services work is challenging and at times exhausting, having stress management skills, a sense of humor, a long-term perspective, and an ability to have fun in the workplace are essential. Self-care is an ethical obligation of clinicians and clinical supervisors. It is in the best interests of clients, clinicians, treatment programs, and the field as a whole that self-care be part of the process for staff and clinicians. In addition to all the above components to self-care, many DBT skills are useful for self-care in the work environment. Some examples are:

• Turtling	• Half-smile	• MEDDSS
• Wise Mind	• Self Soothe 1st Aid Kit	• Broken Record
• Effectively	• Turning the Mind	• GIVE and FAST
• Nonjudgmental	• Ride the Wave	• DEAR WOMAN
• Willingness	• Lemonade	• Radical Acceptance

5. *Diagnosing and seeing deficits and having a strength-based perspective.*

Medical necessity requires that clinical syndromes be diagnosed. Insurance companies, managed care organizations, Medicaid, and Medicare require a diagnosis to authorize payment for services. Many training programs and clinical texts outline symptoms and pathologies, and some mental health and addiction models view problems from a disease perspective. The medical model is pervasive in its focus on deficits and problems.

In recent years, however, a growing contingent has moved away from the deficit perspective to focus on clients' strengths. Many models advocate focusing on healthy development and clients' strengths to empower them to effectively deal with difficulties and stressors. Being strength-based taps into an individual's resiliency. It is an optimistic and hopeful perspective.

Probably a piece of each of these perspectives is useful. Many clients have problems that can be solved, deficits that can be overcome, skills that can be expanded, and strengths that can be improved for the client's own benefit. This often results in an increase in functioning, relationship effectiveness, and life satisfaction. Holding this dialectic helps clinicians and clients to acknowledge that there are strengths and weaknesses in each person. Learning to minimize weaknesses and optimize strengths fosters dialectical thinking and behavior.

6. *Wanting clients to change while not always being patient or positively reinforcing change.*

Clinicians believe in change. Therapy and treatment are all about improvement in the client's lives. Clients may also want things to change, whether that change is in themselves, in others, or in the world around them. Yet the system and clinicians may expect significant change to happen quickly and to be long-lasting. Clients and their families may have similar expectations.

Change does not happen quickly and there is potential for return to old behaviors once change has occurred. The treatment system, clinicians, clients, and their families may be impatient and have unrealistic expectations about how and when change occurs. Of course, there may also be differences of opinion about how, when, and even who will change. Part of the change process is to provide encouragement and rewards for any movement toward positive change. Clinicians use praise, coaching, supporting self-efficacy, and perhaps even incentives. Failing to provide positive reinforcement can result in clients' making little or no change.

Stages of Change (Prochaska, Norcross, and DiClemente, 1994) provides an important framework for understanding where the client is in the change process. Their recommendations for types of interventions depend on the clients' stage of change (SOC) regarding a particular issue. Change is not always a linear, straightforward process. Utilizing the SOC framework can help clients to build motivation for change and empower them to sustain the change over time. For additional suggestions about how to foster change see Motivational Interviewing by William Miller and Stephen Rollnick (2nd Edition, 2002).

STAGES OF CHANGE

PreContemplation

Definition:	Suggested Interventions:
Not being aware of the problem.	• *Observe and Describe*
Doesn't think change is necessary.	• *Moment to Pause*
Wants things to stay the same.	• *Willingness*
	• *Love Dandelions*
	• *ABC*
	• *Relationships Thinking*
	• *Broken Record*

Contemplation

Definition:
Considering options. Open to the idea of change, but is hoping that not much effort will be required. Not ready to make any changes yet.

Suggested Interventions:
- *One Mindfully*
- *Body Scan*
- *Pros & Cons*
- *Turning the Mind*
- *Feeling Not Acting*
- *CARES*
- *Relationship Assumptions*
- *Ignore*

Preparation

Definition:
Has decided to change. Making plans. Can go too slowly or too quickly through this stage.

Suggested Interventions:
- *ONE MIND*
- *Self Soothe First-Aid Kit*
- *Lemonade*
- *Ride the Wave*
- *Interactions in Relationships*

Action

Definition:
Putting the plan into to action. Making changes.

Suggested Interventions:
- *Participate*
- *Be Mindful*
- *OBJECTIVES*
- *Opposite to Emotions*
- *GIVE/FAST*

Maintenance

Definition:
Changes have taken hold. Has stabilized with new lifestyle.

Suggested Interventions:
- *Turtling*
- *Effectively*
- *Self Soothe*
- *Radical Acceptance*
- *MEDDSS*
- *Repairs*
- *4 Horsemen*

Return to Old Behavior/Relapse

Definition:
A return to old thinking, feeling, impulses, and behavior can happen at any stage. Relapse often starts days or weeks before the actual behavior occurs.

Suggested Interventions:
- *Wise Mind*
- *Nonjudgmental*
- *Crisis Survival Network*
- *Half-Smile*
- *BEHAVIORS*
- *DEAR WOMAN*

Clinicians can achieve balance in expecting change by being patient and positively reinforcing efforts to change by utilizing shaping principles or the SOC framework and by assisting clients in increasing their internal motivation for change (Prochaska, Norcross, and DiClemente, 1994). In particular the Decisional Balance Sheet intervention can be very helpful in moving the client forward (Miller & Rollnick, 2002).

DECISIONAL BALANCE SHEET:

Positives for Staying the Same	Negatives of Change
Negatives for Staying the Same	Positives of Change

7. *Being critical of self while being compassionate toward others.*

Much has been written about the importance of compassion and empathy in the therapeutic process and how they facilitate change in clients. Compassion and empathy are qualities that many models of therapy require of clinicians. Some clients display problematic social skills or engage in destructive behaviors, and yet clinicians are able to find ways to attach with these clients as well. Having an understanding, compassionate stance with these clients welcomes them to the therapeutic process so that the work can proceed and change can occur.

The same clinicians, who are able to form these supportive therapeutic alliances, may have very little compassion toward themselves. These clinicians may be critical of their abilities and highlight their weaknesses. They may hold themselves to higher standards of competency or productivity than they hold clients or colleagues to, and when they don't meet these standards they judge themselves negatively. They may tap into their thoughts about being incompetent, a fraud or impostor, or lacking clinical talent. The more they believe that they lack competency the more evidence they can find to support their perspective while at the same time ignoring any data that contradicts it. This creates self-doubt and distress. It may even become a self-fulfilling prophecy.

Balance can be achieved with this dialectic by ensuring that compassion for clients doesn't become enabling, while at the same time appreciating one's own strengths and suspending the need to be so self-critical.

8. *Being committed to professional endeavors and investing in personal life.*

Similar to the self-care dialectic, clinicians may find themselves out of balance and struggling to have both a full personal life and an engaging professional career. Being a human services clinician can be a thankless job at times. There is overwhelming need and insufficient funding for many needed services. Even private practice clinicians may experience tension around client need and limited financial resources. Clinicians may find themselves working very hard and putting in a lot of hours that take most or all of their energy. Many graduate training programs require taking multiple classes at once to achieve immersion in the clinical training process. Clinical training expectations range from part-time experiences of 10–15 hours per week to full-time opportunities that require 50–60 hours per week or even more.

A clinician's personal life, like that of other professionals, may include family, parenting, educational pursuits, religious or spiritual practices, service work, involvement in recovery organizations, and recreational pursuits. Having the time and energy to engage in these activities can be a struggle for the clinician with a full professional life.

Professional obligations tend to outweigh investment in one's personal life. Clinicians may find themselves devoting 90–100% of their focus to their professional activities and practically none to their personal lives. This can lead to frustration, exhaustion, and burnout. Clinicians experiencing burnout may significantly cut back professional obligations or leave the field entirely due to an inability to find an adequate balance with this dialectic.

Clinicians can find balance with this dialectic by having functional boundaries with professional endeavors, developing the ability to leave work at work, and not enabling clients or peers, thus ensuring they have the time and energy to fully participate in their own personal lives. This is another dialectic where clinicians can "walk the talk" to role model for clients as well as to instill resilience in their work.

9. *Being competent while having a lifelong commitment to learning.*

The ethical guidelines for nearly all human services professionals require clinicians to be competent in their professional endeavors. This may include working with a specific population such as children, teenagers, families, or older adults. It can also include competence with particular models or interventions such as CBT, DBT, MI, or Trauma work. The licensure and certification processes are designed to document demonstration of competence in providing clinical services. Before independent practice can be established, professional organizations expect each clinician to display competency with the client populations he intends to treat.

These same professional organizations and licensing boards also charge the clinicians to engage in lifelong learning. This happens through continuing education requirements which vary from 20 to 30 hours of continuing education, on average, per year. There are many ways to engage in continuing education classes: home-study courses, professional conferences, seminars, immersion experiences, summer institutes, webinars, phone seminars, and clinical supervision. In addition to this formal process, many clinicians engage in informal opportunities through reading on their own, participating in book and literature study groups, consultation with peers, and other opportunities.

This dialectic is balanced when clinicians can establish a minimum competency in the work while engaging in ongoing professional development and maintaining a commitment to using state-of-the-art models and interventions.

10. *Wanting to be good at DBT before being ready to invest the time and energy to do so.*

Clinicians often comment that they were already doing DBT but did not know it. DBT has many CBT components, however, DBT is designed to require teaching skills explicitly and then holding clients accountable to practice, use, and demonstrate them in the therapy room and in their lives. DBT is not just about the skills, it is also about having a dialectical perspective, staying in balance in the therapeutic relationship, and using the DBT skills themselves in the work. So it is possible to start using some DBT skills right after taking a seminar or reading about it, however, there is more to this model.

Building competency with DBT takes time, energy, and dedication. Individuals truly interested in implementing DBT in a comprehensive way will need to read about the model, practice it in their own lives, engage in professional consultation and supervision, and perhaps even invest in an immersion training experience. There is so much to this model that it is possible to spend months or even a few years integrating DBT into one's clinical practice.

CLINICIAN DIALECTICS CONCLUSION

Similar to clients, clinicians experience a variety of dialectics in their professional endeavors, and they, too, will benefit from being able to balance these dialectics. They will build resilience in their work lives and improve their effectiveness as well as take an opportunity to "walk the talk," which builds credibility with clients. Gaining this insight on the experiences of being in and out of balance can show the clinician some of the challenges and opportunities that clients face as part of balancing dialectics.

THERAPEUTIC ALLIANCE DIALECTICS

1. Acceptance and change

2. Centeredness and flexibility

3. Nurturing and benevolently demanding

4. Emotional intimacy and boundaries

5. Unconditional positive regard with limits and natural and logical consequences

6. Skill enhancement and self-acceptance

7. Problem solving and problem acceptance

8. Self-efficacy and asking for help

9. Irreverent and validating communication

10. Immediate needs, short-term goals, and long-term outcomes

These dialectics are dynamic interactions between the client, the clinician and the treatment system.

1. *Acceptance and change.*

This is a major dialectic in DBT. On one hand, acceptance of the client, his situation, the clinician, and the system is useful. This is a place to have understanding and compassion for the client, oneself, and the community. One part of this dialectic can be seen in the DBT philosophy that clients are doing the best they can, given their internal strengths and weakness and their environmental experiences. Clients' thoughts and behaviors are a result of what they have learned about themselves, others, and the world around them. When life is threatening and unsafe, it makes sense that clients engage in significant controlling behavior. When life is very hard most or all of the time, being suicidal makes logical sense to the clients experiencing it.

Acceptance that clients are doing the best they can is valid for both client and clinician. Acceptance of the clinician's strengths and weaknesses, and his own learning history is also part of the process. While it isn't appropriate for clinicians to self-disclose to this extent, it is important for clinicians to have acceptance of themselves.

This also applies to treatment systems. There are certainly many imperfections in most local and national treatment systems. There are limitations and resiliency within the system. Overall, acceptance of the realities of the client, clinician, and system is useful...and only half the story.

The other half is that change is required. The only valid option for clients is to work hard, learn DBT skills, and change. Change empowers clients to experience improvement, hope, and optimism. Change is often a difficult process. It takes hard work, dedication, frustration tolerance, the ability to make mistakes, and staying the course. Sometimes the best learning comes from negative experiences and disappointments. Most clients have tried other things before, but since previous therapy, reading self-help books, and other strategies have been insufficient or even made things worse, DBT may be the most promising option.

DBT requires a balance of acceptance and expecting change. This can be facilitated by the clinician by providing support and normalizing the client's experiences while engaging in well-timed interventions that are designed to move the client forward. Using the SOC framework (see above) will assist in this process.

2. *Centeredness and flexibility.*

Centeredness is about being grounded in the midst of the pain and trauma the client has experienced. This pain and trauma may have happened in childhood, adulthood, or both. The therapy process may entail bearing witness to this pain and trauma. The clinician's ability to make therapy safe and supportive will facilitate this process. Clinicians need to be able to sit with clients as they explore their experiences, losses, grief, and disappointments while finding the strength to be effective in their lives in the here and now. The ability to stay present in the face of enormous pain and emotional intensity is an important clinical competency.

Flexibility is about meeting clients where they are and focusing on what they want to work on. Flexibility may be about setting aside the agenda for one session or letting the client "off the hook" from practicing the skills.

Centeredness is also about having appropriate boundaries. Appropriate boundaries include emotional, physical, financial, and interpersonal boundaries. Clients will increase their effectiveness when they work within appropriate boundaries. While some boundaries can be flexible, being too flexible by not enforcing the rules may allow for the client to continue in their nonproductive behavior.

Being out of balance with flexibility or centeredness can look like being rigid or too loose. The challenge is to do a little bit of both without doing too much of either. This can be accomplished by staying in the moment, holding the boundaries, and bending and flexing therapeutically.

3. *Nurturing and benevolently demanding.*

Nurturing is about being a coach, teacher, or mentor to the client. Here the clinician provides positive reinforcement for anything that supports the client in staying the course with therapy and integrating DBT skills. Nurturing is about providing support and understanding for the client when he is frustrated, experiencing a setback, or feeling like a failure.

Benevolently demanding is part of effective parenting as well as the basis of the educational system. It is about having high and achievable expectations. Goals and expectations should be set high enough that clients need to stretch and grow while not being so hard that clients become frustrated and give up...or so easy that clients become bored and give up. Having supportive and challenging expectations fosters development. Clients may grow and improve in ways they may not have imagined possible.

This dialectic is about working hard and giving the client credit for the work they have accomplished. It is also about being flexible at times by taking a break or slowing down. Balance can be achieved when clinicians provide positive reinforcement for progress made while pushing the client forward to live in more effective ways.

4. *Emotional intimacy and boundaries.*

Therapy is an emotionally intimate experience in many cases. Clients are exposing their vulnerabilities, sharing their deepest fears, and grappling with their own imperfections. They explore their internal realities and environmental experiences. They may have a wide range of emotions in the therapy room from despair to anger. There may be tears and tension. Depending on the therapy model, learning about emotions, working through the pain, and learning not to act on emotions are part of the therapeutic process. In the midst of these emotional expressions the therapeutic relationship is intensified. Client and clinician become closer. Clinicians may experience increased attachment and appreciation for the client. The safety and groundedness of the clinician provides the opportunity for the client to go even deeper emotionally on a regular basis.

While the work is emotionally intimate it is still important to maintain boundaries. Therapy is not an interaction of peers. Clients are seeking help whether they come voluntarily or are mandated to treatment. They share their understanding of their life, struggles, and painful experiences, and replicate their relationships in the therapy room. The clinician, however, is in this relationship as a professional. He is there to be a guide and mentor, not to share his own struggles and painful experiences. As the relationship gets deeper and more intimate clients and clinicians may drift into looser boundaries. This is a slippery slope that can lead to confusion, boundary crossings, and, in its extreme forms, inappropriate behavior.

It is the clinician's responsibility to maintain balance with this dialectic. This dialectic can be balanced with the clinician meeting his own needs outside of the therapy room, using supervision and consultation, knowing when he is in need of therapy, and having a thorough informed consent.

Informed consent outlines what happens in therapy and what doesn't. While this is a written contract that is created at the beginning of therapy and it can also be an ongoing understanding about what is appropriate in therapy and what isn't. Clients haven't always grown up in functional families with healthy boundaries, so it makes sense that they will push and resist limits set by the clinician. As the professional, it is the clinician's responsibility to maintain boundaries while not becoming unnecessarily rigid.

5. *Unconditional positive regard with limits and natural and logical consequences.*

Unconditional positive regard, in which the clinician forms an empathic relationship with the client, is a major component of humanistic psychology. The clinician accepts the client for who he is, rather than viewing the client's behavior as defining who the client is. Part of this therapeutic process is to be nonjudgmental with clients. It is about not assigning a value to the client as good or bad even though his behavior may be good or bad.

Behavior provokes natural and logical consequences that can be positive or negative. Clients' completing homework and demonstrating DBT skills in their lives should receive the natural and logical consequences of praise, encouragement, and the expectation to learn additional skills. When a client doesn't practice skills, the natural and logical consequences could be role-playing the skill in session, discussing why the skill was not practiced, and letting the client know that the expectation is to practice the skill. Not showing up or derailing the therapy may require setting expectations, holding the client accountable, and perhaps even behavioral contracts. With severe behavior such as acting out in the office, being threatening, or destroying property, terminating the therapy relationship may be the most appropriate action. There is a fine line between natural and logical consequences and punishment, which is defined by the level of severity and whether there is a component of acting out negative feelings on the part of the clinician. This can happen when the clinician's countertransference goes unchecked and his reactions become an expression of frustration, irritation, and anger at the client. The other extreme would be not applying natural and logical consequences when they are appropriate and warranted.

Balancing this dialectic requires forming relationships with clients without enabling them and applying natural and logical consequences in a consistent manner. Consistency is a dialectic. It is imperfect: it will wax and wane. Clinicians must do their best to be consistent and still allow for inconsistency to be part of the process. Clinicians are encouraged to keep their codependency in check and see both the positives and negatives in the therapeutic relationship and in the client's behaviors as well as their own.

6. *Skill enhancement and self-acceptance.*

Some clients are interested in increasing their skills. They spend a lot of time and energy in this pursuit. They have read many self-help books, they spend hours on the Internet, and they watch the media clinicians like Dr. Phil. They listen to advice and watch for new trends in life, career, and family perspectives. These clients believe that their problems will be solved when they find the next idea, way of life, or spiritual or philosophical perspective. They are searching to find the solution outside themselves. While in this pursuit they don't give themselves credit for the strengths and skills they do have. They don't maintain awareness of the ways in which they have grown and improved their lives.

There are other clients who are all about self-acceptance. They believe that they are fine and don't need to change in any way. If a change needs to happen it must be about other people. These clients have personal philosophies that sound like: "It's my way or the highway," "You're either with me or against me," or "Love me or leave me alone." Unfortunately there is erroneous logic with this position. There is always something new to learn or to improve. For many clients there may be considerable room for improvement, even with an adequately functioning individual. In addition to this logic being erroneous it may also be arrogant. Clients with this perspective may be disrespectful, aggressive, and perhaps even ignore the rights of others.

Either of these two perspectives can benefit from a little of the other to achieve balance. Clinicians can help each of these clients by helping them see that a little more acceptance, or enhancement of their skills, will be useful. Adding the opposite of the initial focus will empower clients to be more effective so that they can build a life worth living. Balance can be achieved in the therapeutic relationship by the clinician helping clients to be aware that they can improve and increase their skills while also learning to accept themselves and their lives.

7. *Problem solving and problem acceptance.*

There are times when problems can be solved. Clients can figure out solutions: they can ask family, friends, and clinicians for advice or ideas. They can use their past experiences to figure out what to do. They can advocate for themselves. They can research what to do on the Internet or at the library. They can take action to solve the problem, and they can be curious about trying other things if the first thing they try doesn't work. This can be a very effective process and yet there also problems that can't be solved.

When a problem can't be solved or resolved in a satisfactory manner accepting the problem may make sense. Sometimes clients learn that they don't always get it their way no matter how hard they work, ask for help, or apologize. Clients' accepting that there are things they cannot control is an important step in being empowered to invest where they do have control. Clients can also be out of balance with this part of the dialectic when they sink into passivity. They may think that nearly everything is out of their control. Taking a victim or martyr stance may be a natural part of this imbalance. But even when problems can't be solved clients can maintain control over their thoughts, feelings, and behavior.

A variation of this dialectic is regulating and tolerating emotions. Clients have many opportunities to learn to cope with, manage, and regulate their emotions—this may be an everyday occurrence. By comparison, there are times when the only thing that can be done is to tolerate emotions. This may be true with strong emotions and those that last a long time such as grief. There may be no way to resolve the loss that the client is grieving. Perhaps all they can do is tolerate and accept the grief for a while. It is possible for a client to get stuck in his grief and stay in it too long. In these situations the client will eventually need to move away from the grief and into living life in the here and now, with the loss as part of his history.

Clinicians can help clients to stay in balance with this dialectic by alternating active strategies with acceptance perspectives. In particular, Lemonade, Willingness, and Radical Acceptance might be particularly helpful with this dialectic.

8. *Self-efficacy and asking for help.*

Some clients live their lives as if they can do everything themselves. They may have learned not to trust others. Family and friends may have disappointed them in the past when they didn't help or made things worse than they needed to be. Having learned to be self-contained because others aren't reliable, these clients attempt to be their only resource. There are probably many things for which clients can rely on themselves as their self-efficacy becomes more pervasive; however, there is a limit to what any one person can do on their own. Clinicians may encounter this situation when a client won't talk about what is difficult or challenging and won't take advice or direction. Being able to ask for help when it will be useful and to choose someone who is able to help are necessary competencies to be in balance with this dialectic.

At the other extreme of this dialectic are clients who ask for help even when they can do things themselves. These clients become dependent on others when they don't need to be. They look for others to give direction and solve their problems even when they have the skills and resources to take care of themselves in many ways. Clinicians see evidence of this imbalance when the client can't seem to make decisions, requires concrete directions from the clinician, or makes excessive requests for help on basic issues.

Clinicians can work toward balance in the therapeutic relationship with this dialectic by helping clients learn that they can effectively take care of themselves and manage their lives while knowing when, how, and whom to ask for help.

9. *Irreverent and validating communication.*

Irreverent communication is about having fun, displaying a sense of humor, and not taking oneself too seriously. Therapists can poke fun at themselves to model that clients can laugh at themselves and not always be so intense. Irreverent communication seeks to disrupt crisis-building behavior. It responds to the most outrageous or worrisome part of what the client is saying and takes it a step further. This illustrates that the client's position is extreme and perhaps illogical. Having fun and a sense of humor in therapy can be helpful and yet it can be disrespectful or passive-aggressive. It is crucial that the clinician use this communication style with skill.

By comparison, validating communication is supportive. It acknowledges the reality of the client's life. Many clients grow up hearing that their thoughts, feelings, and behaviors are wrong, inaccurate, and unacceptable, and in environments and relationships that invalidate them. They learn that they should be different from who they are, which isn't really possible.

Therapy and treatment should validate the client, accepting the reality of his life while helping him to see other perspectives. Clinicians can achieve balance in the therapeutic relationship with this dialectic by ensuring that each session has a good amount of both irreverent and validating communication. This communication should be a two-way street with both the clinician and client giving and getting this type of process.

10. *Immediate needs, short-term goals, and long-term outcomes.*

This is a three-way dialectic. The client, clinician, and therapy can balance immediate needs, short-term goals, and long-term outcomes. This dialectic is a bit like juggling. Attention and effort needs to be made periodically in each domain. Being out of balance with this dialectic can lead to progress being made in one of these areas, but perhaps at the cost of the expectations in other domains. Clients may have difficulty learning how to stay grounded with each of these domains without becoming overwhelmed and feeling immobilized.

Clinicians can help achieve balance with this dialectic by empowering clients to meet their immediate needs while working at their short-term goals as well as keeping an eye on their ultimate desired outcome. All the preceding therapeutic alliance dialectics can contribute to the success of balance in this dialectic.

THERAPEUTIC DIALECTICS

Being out of balance in one or more of these dialectics can cause the therapy to lose its forward momentum. When things stop moving forward or there is an impasse the therapy may be out of balance. It is the responsibility of the clinician to maintain balance in the therapeutic relationship.

DIALECTICAL CONCLUSIONS

There are many opportunities for balance and imbalance for the client, the clinician, and in the interactions between clients and clinicians. Balance can be experienced internally or in interactions. Balance will facilitate the clinical work and foster the relationship for the benefit of both individuals.

Balance is imperfect. It doesn't have to be exactly in the center. It is possible to be in balance while still being a bit askew to one side or the other. It is also possible to vacillate between one side and the other, while still being in balance.

The above lists are only a sampling of dialectics that might be present for the client, clinician, or in the therapeutic relationship. Some questions that clinicians might ask themselves are on the next page.

1. What additional dialectics would improve clients' experiences?

    _____

    _____

    _____

2. How can clients get in balance with these dialectics?

    _____

    _____

    _____

3. What dialectics do clinicians experience in their work?

    _____

    _____

    _____

4. How can clinicians get in balance with these dialectics?

    _____

    _____

    _____

5. What dialectics are present in the therapeutic relationship?

    _____

    _____

    _____

6. How can balance be achieved with these dialectics in the relationship?

    _____

    _____

    _____

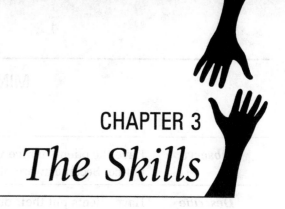

CHAPTER 3
The Skills

DBT consists of four content areas: Mindfulness, Distress Tolerance, Emotional Regulation, and Interpersonal Effectiveness. A fifth module, the Middle Path, is for teenagers and their families. It doesn't have its own set of skills, but pulls skills from the other four modules to instill balance in families (Miller, Rathus.& Linehan, 2006).

There are a number of traditional, or "classic," DBT skills created by Dr. Linehan (Linehan 1993a; Linehan, 1993b). There are also innovative skills created by other authors, including the one producing this text (Marra, 2004; Moonshine, 2007; Spradlin, 2003). These skills have been created through dynamic interactions between clinicians and clients, tying the skills to the philosophy and precepts of DBT, and relating DBT skills to existing evidence-based practices and what the research says works.

On the following pages are a variety of DBT skills. These are not the only skills that can be used when teaching clients. Clinicians can find additional skills in other texts, on the Internet, and in professional articles. Clinicians can also create their own skills. One framework for creating your own skills would be:

- Determine which module you are developing skills for.
- Take into consideration cultural values, developmental milestones, and clients' worldview.
- Outline how the skill will facilitate balanced dialectics.
- Make it relevant to your clients.
- Appeal to visual, auditory, and kinesthetic learners.
- Be responsive to client attention span.
- Utilize multiple media.
- Make learning fun, interesting, creative, and relevant.
- Learn from the wisdom of your clients.
- On the following pages is the DBT Skills Crosswalk.

MINDFULNESS

Classic

Observe	Have the clients notice what is going on around and inside themselves. Just notice. Become aware of things in this one moment.
Describe	Have clients put their observations into concrete, specific terms, while being as nonjudgmental as possible. Clients can describe a thing non-judgmentally by saying that it is unacceptable, that they don't like it, that it is painful, or that they hate it. Judgmental descriptions would assign value to themselves or others. Examples: That person is an idiot, I am terrible and deserve to be in pain, or it's hopeless, I will never be good enough.
Participate	By observing what is going on inside and around them and describing things concretely, clients are able to fully participate in their lives in a mindful way. They can participate completely in each activity they engage in.
Non-Judgmental	<ul><li>Suspending evaluations about self and others.</li><li>Judging behavior as right or wrong, good or bad, but not judging the person engaging in the behavior. Behavior can generate natural and logical consequences, but we don't label the person engaging in it.</li><li>Describing things concretely.</li><li>Liking or disliking things.</li><li>Holding values that are beliefs or ethics, not judgments.</li></ul>
One-Mindfully	Teach clients to do one thing at a time. Each activity or behavior in which they engage needs to be done mindfully, and then they can move onto to the next activity or behavior, still dedicating themselves to each thing individually at a time. For some clients this may mean slowing down, which may be more effective than the pace at which they are living. Other clients may be able to live a fast-paced life while being one-mindful.
Effectively	<ul><li>Working with clients to be as effective as possible in their lives.</li><li>Helping them to see what is more effective and avoid less effective strategies and behaviors.</li><li>Avoid judgmental words such as better, worse, good, or bad.</li></ul>
Wise Mind	Balancing Rational Mind and Emotional Mind to create Wise Mind. Clients are able to be more mindful and effective when they use both Rational and Emotional Mind. Be sure that clients aren't judging Rational Mind as good and Emotional Mind as bad. By being in Wise Mind, clients are in balance and have all their senses, ways of knowing, and skills at their disposal to manage their lives effectively and to act in their own best interest.

MINDFULNESS

Innovative

Moment to Pause   This skill teaches clients to take a quick moment to check in with themselves on the inside, in their environment, and their interactions. By being grounded inside and around themselves they are able to make decisions and behave in ways that are in their best interest.

By taking a moment to pause, clients can stop a destructive or problematic behavior and replace it with a DBT skill. This is a simple but essential skill in reaching the goal of building a life worth living.

Square Breathing   When clients take a few deep breaths it creates a moment to pause. It also results in getting more oxygen to their muscles and brains, so they may feel a bit less tense and think a bit more clearly. It also provides another opportunity for the client to disengage from destructive or problematic behavior and utilize another skill.

1. Breathe in while counting to four.
2. Hold it for four seconds.
3. Then exhale while counting to four.
4. Repeat four times.

Mindful Eating   This exercise is about being fully present in the ritual of eating. It asks clients to experience the complexity and richness of eating. Clients may find themselves eating at their desk at work, in the car, or in front of the TV. While this may serve a purpose, ask them to find 3–4 times a week to eat mindfully.

Eating mindfully requires that the clients focus just on eating. They use their senses to appreciate the food. They chew each bite fully. By doing so, they will eat less food in the 15–20 minutes it takes to feel full. While being mindful, hopefully they will notice the sensation of fullness and satiation. Chewing each bite fully also produces more saliva which is one of the most effective enzymes in digestion, enabling food to be digested more completely.

ONE MIND   <u>O</u>ne thing at a time

<u>N</u>ow, be in the here and now

<u>E</u>nvironment, grounded in it

<u>M</u>oment, be present in this one moment

<u>I</u>ncrease senses to be firmly in the here and now

<u>N</u>on-Judgmental of self and others

<u>D</u>escribe things in concrete, specific terms

This acronym helps clients stay present in the moment inside and around them.

MINDFULNESS

Innovative

Body Scan
Taking a few moments, have clients focus on their bodies. Clients can do this with their eyes closed or open. They can do it almost anywhere and several times a day. This exercise brings the client into the here and now and may also put their pain in perspective by making space for comfort and neutral sensations. Provide instructions to the clients by first asking clients to go inside themselves. Here are some suggested instructions to give to clients.

- Notice any pain, discomfort, and tension you are feeling
- Just notice it, don't do anything about it
- Notice relaxation, comfort, and feeling at ease
- Also become aware of neutral sensations
- Take another moment to be with yourself on the inside
- Now become aware of yourself on the outside
- Notice your feet on the ground
- Become of aware of the environment with all five of your senses
- Lighting, temperature, sound, perhaps smell and taste
- Become of aware of people around you, closeness and distance. Even if they are in another room or building, image their proximity
- One more moment on the outside, the inside and come back

Be Mindful
This skill asks clients to be mindful of one or two things. The client pays attention to practicing a specific skill or staying in the moment. Ask clients to Be Mindful of self care, having healthy fun, and connection to support system.

Turtling
Clients use a variety of strategies to take care of themselves, just like turtles.

- Retreating inside themselves and then reemerging when it is safe.
- Going slowly and methodically, being thoughtful about how to invest time, energy, and attention.
- Using their hard outer shells to let things roll off their backs. This is a great way to deflect the judgments of others.
- Being adaptive; turtles are able to live in water and on land.
- Persistently self-righting. When turtles get turned over, they use their weight and environment to get themselves right-side up and back in balance. It may take a few hours or even a couple of days, but when life turns turtles upside down, they work hard to right themselves and get back in balance.
- Although they aren't aggressive animals, turtles will protect themselves when absolutely necessary through snapping or biting.

Turtles are very important symbols in many cultures or communities such as Native American and Hindu. Turtling will also resonate with kids and teenagers, because of Teenage Mutant Ninja Turtles.

DISTRESS TOLERANCE

Classic

Exploring Pros & Cons

This skill explores:

- Pros of having crisis
- Cons of not having crisis
- Pros of not having crisis
- Cons of having crisis

Pros of having Crisis or Stress	Cons of not having Crisis or Stress
Cons of having Crisis or Stress	Pros of not having Crisis or Stress

Most of us would put an emphasis on the last two, but it is enormously helpful to explore the first two.

What does the client get out of having crises?

- Extra attention
- Held less responsible
- Adrenaline rush
- Scaring others

Help the client meet their needs in a more direct, effective way so they don't need crises.

What are the downsides to not having crises?

- It's boring
- Having to do all those mundane things like clean the house
- Less support from family and friends
- Accepting full responsibility

Assist the client in building the skills to successfully balance responsibility, chores, and expectations with fun, enjoyment, and relationships.

Self Soothe

Have the clients self-soothe with all five of their senses: sight, sound, smell, taste, and touch. The caveat of this skill is that if they overly self-soothe with a particular sense then they skip that sense. For example if the client overeats, then taste is not the sense to self-soothe with.

DISTRESS TOLERANCE

Classic

Turning the Mind This one teaches clients that they are in the driver's seat with their mind. This includes thoughts, feelings, impulses, and even behavior.

Clients can identify which road they are driving on. They can choose to stay on the same road or they can make a left turn changing their thoughts, feelings, impulses, or behavior. They can make a right turn which would take their thoughts, feelings, impulses, or behaviors in a different direction. They can also make a U-turn and start over. It is also possible for clients to stop driving for a while and take a break.

Observe Breathing This exercise orients client to their breath. Ask clients to spend a few moments paying attention to their breath. One way this is helpful is as a distraction from the crisis or stressful situation. It also can have a calming effect by providing more oxygen to the mind and body, reducing anxiety or distressing bodily sensations. Here are some ways you can direct clients to use this skill:

- Inhale while counting to 5 slowly
- Let the breath out will counting to 5 slowly
- Repeat 5 times

- Take a deep breath while taking one long stride
- Let out the breath while taking one long stride
- Repeat 3 times

- Take long slow breaths in and out while imagining relaxing on a beach or at home under the covers. Do this for 90 seconds.

- For every distressing thought or painful sensation complete a full deep breath in and out.

Willingness Willingness exercises are helpful in the middle of a crisis. Clients can practice willingness to accept reality, a bad day, things not going their way, or to accept that they can't control others and the world around them. Willingness is open and accepting. It is life-enhancing, energy generating and relationship enhancing. By comparison, willfulness is acting like a 2 year old. Wanting what we want even when it isn't in our best interest or does us harm. Willfulness is exhausting, harms relationships, and reduces quality of life.

DISTRESS TOLERANCE

Classic

ACCEPTS	Have clients distract themselves with: **A**ctivities **C**ompassion **C**hoices **E**motions **P**ushing Away **T**houghts **S**ensations
IMPROVE	This acronym provides a series of things for the clients to focus on that will distract them from a crisis or stressful situation. Clients can take their time with this one, which will give their nervous system time to settle down. **I**magery **M**eaning **P**rayer **R**elaxation **O**ne-Mindfully **V**acation **E**ncouragement
Half Smile	Have the clients find something in their day or in their lives that can give them a genuine half-smile. It can be: • A good cup of coffee • Blue sky • Payday • A long weekend coming up • A pleasant memory • The joy on child's face When a client has a half-smile, they are a bit more relaxed in their face, neck, and shoulders. People respond differently to someone with a smile than to someone who is angry or upset. If the client is treated nicely because they are smiling that might improve their day a little bit more.
Radical Acceptance	• The Serenity Prayer • Clients can control themselves in terms of their thoughts, feelings and actions. • Clients don't have control over what happens around them or what others do. • The clients effectively focus their attention and energy on what they can control and change: themselves.

DISTRESS TOLERANCE

Innovative

Crisis Survival Network	It is important for everyone to have a crisis survival network. Hopefully your clients have one and you are not the only one on it. Educate your clients about who is helpful to have on their list and people who make things worse. Having as many people as possible on the list, and using them flexibly, are key to making this skill most useful.
Keeping It In Perspective	Ask the clients if this is the worst crisis they have ever had to deal with. Typically they will answer this affirmatively. If so, you create a metaphor that this is the marathon of crises and all of their other crises and difficulties have been in training. The clients are now in the best shape of their lives. They are well experienced and they can definitely deal with this crisis effectively.
Self Soothe First Aid Kit	This one can be quite creative. The client puts together a kit that is self soothing. It can be on their computer, in their purse/wallet, or desk drawer. It can be a box that they decorate and fill with things that are soothing for them. Things in the self soothe 1st Aid Kit have to be effective and not harmful in any way. An alternative way to talk about this skill is to call it a tool kit, not a 1st aid kit.
OBJECTIVES	Clients can use this acronym to effectively deal with difficult experiences.

1. <u>O</u>ne thing at a time
2. <u>B</u>e effective
3. Avoid <u>J</u>udgments
4. Cope with <u>E</u>motions
5. Consider <u>C</u>onsequences
6. Take <u>T</u>ime
7. Use <u>I</u>ntrospection
8. Act consistently with <u>V</u>alues
9. Focus on desired <u>E</u>ndings
10. Balance <u>S</u>hort-term and long-term goals

SPECIFIC PATHS	This acronym helps clients stay on path to build the life they want for themselves.

1. What is my <u>S</u>upreme Concern?
2. <u>P</u>ractice my skills
3. Focus my <u>E</u>nergy and <u>C</u>oncentration
4. <u>I</u> can be effective
5. Have <u>F</u>aith
6. Consider what is <u>I</u>mportant
7. Have <u>C</u>ourage and <u>P</u>atience
8. Pay <u>A</u>ttention
9. Complete <u>T</u>asks
10. Be <u>H</u>umble and have <u>S</u>ensitivity

EMOTIONAL REGULATION

Classic

ABC	Using this acronym helps clients to achieve balance in the face of difficult situations. When the client is having a bad day or something unpleasant occurs, they can use this skill to remind themselves of positive things they are good at and use strategies that they have prepared for just such occasions. **A**ccumulate Positives **B**uild Mastery **C**ope Ahead
MEDDSS	This skill is all about self-care. Self-care dramatically enhances our emotional well being: **M**astery **E**xercise **D**iet **D**rugs (Take prescription drugs as directed but not illicit ones) **S**leep **S**pirituality
Love Dandelions	This skill provides clients with the opportunity to accept themselves or to love their shadow selves. Clients build an awareness and acceptance of parts of themselves that they dislike or find unattractive. There are some things they can't change about themselves, but by being aware of them they can minimize damage and distress.
Opposite to Emotions	First ask the client what emotion they have a lot of that is problematic or troublesome. Ask the clients to be mindfully present with the strong emotions, but not act on them. Ask the clients to identify the opposite emotion to the strong emotion. Then ask the client when they notice the opposite emotion. Have the client identify 4–6 things that they can do on any given day that brings the opposite emotion into their awareness. After this has been established, give the client the assignment that whenever they are feeling the strong emotion, to hold it in their awareness and actively engage in activities that bring the opposite emotion to their awareness as well.

EMOTIONAL REGULATION

Innovative

Lemonade out of Lemons	This skill is about having clients refocus their weaknesses and problematic thinking and behavior into strengths.
	This happens when a client takes the skills and strengths they do have, but may be using in a way that causes harm or problems in their lives. They can take these skills and strengths and focus them differently in their lives.
	For example, an identity thief who becomes a security expert; a car thief who works with police and insurance companies to reduce auto theft; the drug addict who gets into recovery and becomes an addictions counselor.
	With this skill, clients learn they don't have to start over. They learn that while some changes may be required, they don't have to be overwhelmed with trying to be completely different.
Feeling not Acting	Feeling a strong impulse or emotion is not the same as acting on it. This would be two steps. Clients can use their Moment to Pause to identify and feel an impulse or urge. They can choose to engage in the impulse, use a skill to manage it, or tolerate it while doing nothing.
Ride the Wave	This skill uses the metaphor that the tide comes and goes, but it is always with us just like our emotions and strong impulses. Some days are stormy and chaotic while other days are calmer.
	While it might feel like a particular emotional state might last forever or that this is the last feeling the client will ever have, it will eventually shift and change into the next emotion.
	A visualization or artwork exercise could be useful. Direct the client to imagine that they are riding the wave of their emotions. This can be done with surfing, snowboarding, skiing, or skateboarding. It is a lot more fun to do this when it's intense than when it's calm. And to do it well, the client has to be fully in the moment. This skill seems to resonate with teenagers and young adults.

EMOTIONAL REGULATION

Innovative

Build Positive Emotions

The client can balance out negative emotions and experiences by increasing positive emotions and experiences.

Short Term: Do pleasant things that are possible now.

Long term: Make changes in your life so that positive events will occur more often. Build a "life worth living."

1. Work toward goals:
   - Make a list of positive events you want.
   - List small steps toward goals.
   - Take the first step.

2. Attend to relationships:
   - Repair old relationships.
   - Reach out for new relationships.
   - Work on current relationships.

3. Avoid avoiding:
   - Avoid giving up.
   - Effectively and actively problem solve.
   - Do things that are necessary.

Getting to Know Emotions

Have the client explore the following process:

Environmental precipitants. Determine what happened in the environment just prior to your current emotional state.

Identify emotions. Identify and describe your emotions.

Experience in the body. Identify and describe bodily experience of emotions.

Cognitions related to the emotions. Identify and describe the thoughts you are having about your emotions.

Behavior. Identify the behavior that you have engaged in, or have urges to engage in, as a result of your emotional state.

Aftermath. Explore the aftermath of the situation. How did you feel? What happened? What were the positive and negative consequences? What went well? What have you learned? What might you do differently next time?

EMOTIONAL REGULATION

Innovative

Exploring Your Emotions

Assumptions. What assumptions are you making about your feelings, yourself, others, and the world around you?

Counteracting the assumption. How can you counteract or ignore these assumptions?

Notice change in emotion. Identify and describe how your emotional state changes.

Non-judgmental. Apply your non-judgmental skills, both for you and others.

Future Tripping. Evaluate if you are future-tripping; identify and describe.

Challenge tripping. How can you challenge or ignore future-tripping.

One-mindful. Be mindful; be completely present in this one moment.

Meaning about me. What meaning does this emotional state have to you?

Challenge the meaning. Contrast or challenge this meaning to you. Think about how this might be related to the earlier assumption.

Non-judgmental. Once again, apply your non-judgmental skills to yourself and others.

Change Body. Change your posture and energy level. Notice change in emotional state.

Facial Expression. Change your facial expression. Notice change in emotional state.

Change Behaviors. Change your behaviors and activities. Notice change in emotional state.

EMOTIONAL REGULATION

Innovative

CARES   This acronym is short, making it easy to remember. This skill will be useful for clients who need to modulate their arousal response.

Calm, coached practice
Arousal monitoring
Relaxation and rest
Emotions in the environment
Sleep an effective amount

TRUST   This acronym is short, which makes it easy to remember. The client who will benefit from this skill comes across as scary or intimidating without being aware of it.

Trust yourself.
Redirect impulses and urges
Use your skills to be effective
Seen, act consistently on how you want others to see you.
Tame your emotions and reactions

EMOTIONS   This acronym is concrete and straightforward which is useful for some clients.

Exposure to emotions
Mindful of current emotions
Outline a plan to deal with emotions
Take opposite action
Increase positive experiences
Obstacles and plan to overcome them
Notice what is going on
Support system

BEHAVIOR   This is another acronym. This one is useful for clients who want to focus on healing versus hurting behavior or those who are strongly connected with a value system.

Use effective **B**ehavior
Be grounded in the **E**nvironment
Do things that are **H**ealing not Hurting
Act in my best interest
Be consistent with my **V**alues
Imagine getting through difficulties
Focus on the desired **O**utcome
Reinforce my successes

If the client doesn't like a particular letter, they can change it to something else as long as it is effective in being prosocial and well-adjusted.

INTERPERSONAL EFFECTIVENESS

Classic

Broken Record	The client practices being a broken record with themselves. They keep coming back to their needs and wants.
Ignore	Ignore self-judgments and judgments of others
Turn the Tables	Be reciprocal. Do things for other people.
GIVE	This skill is designed to provide the clients with capacities to improve and sustain relationships in healthy ways.

<u>G</u>entle in relationships
<u>I</u>nterest in others
<u>V</u>alidate
<u>E</u>asy Manner

FAST	Self-respect is the goal of this skill. This skill helps clients who are out of balance with codependency or focus on others to also focus on themselves.

<u>F</u>air to self
<u>A</u>pologize less
<u>S</u>tick to values
<u>T</u>ruthful with self

DEAR WOMAN or MAN	This skill is used to accomplish a task or meet an objective. Based on the client's gender I teach them either WOMAN or MAN.

<u>D</u>escribe what is wanted
<u>E</u>ncourage others to help
<u>A</u>sk for what is wanted
<u>R</u>einforce others

<u>W</u>illingness
<u>O</u>bserve
<u>M</u>indful
<u>A</u>ppear Confident
<u>N</u>egotiate

INTERPERSONAL EFFECTIVENESS

Innovative

Relationship Thinking	This skill is about couples and families using dialectical thinking rather than dichotomous thinking.

Dichotomous thinking to avoid:

- Always
- Never
- All or nothing
- Black or white
- This or that
- With me or against me

Dialectical thinking to increase:

- Both/and
- Positive and negative feelings
- Thoughts and feelings
- Shades of gray
- Needs and wants
- Self and others
- Talking and listening
- Balance

Relationship Assumptions	This skill puts the dialectical philosophy into couples' or families' language.

1. Both of us are doing the best we can
2. Both of us can be more effective
3. Both of us want to be more effective
4. Both of have to be more effective, try harder, and apply our skills
5. Neither of us caused all of the problems in our relationship, and we both have to work together to solve them

INTERPERSONAL EFFECTIVENESS

Innovative

Relationship Mindfulness

Clients can apply mindfulness to their relationships:

- Identify generalizations
- Describe assumptions
- Suspend judgments
- Avoid jumping to conclusions
- Empower self, don't defeat self
- Use One-Mindfulness
- Be non-judgmental
- Participate effectively

Interactions in Relationships

This skill helps clients to be in the moment and to interact effectively with family, friends, and others. Below is a list steps that clients can use:

- Observe and Describe the interaction
- Be Mindful of emotions
- Engage in opposite behaviors when useful
- Remember to breathe
- Take a Non-Judgmental stance
- Use assertive communication
- Show self-respect and respect for others
- Develop frustration tolerance

By using this skill clients will experience improved communication, interactions, and more ability to sustain relationships in a variety of contexts.

Dealing with Difficult People

- Describe your relationship
- Describe quality of relationship
- Explore your particular sensitivity to this relationship
- Participate in improving this relationship
- Identify and overcome obstacles to improvement

The Most Difficult

Rate the difficulty, identify feelings, minimize judgments, and engage in effective interactions.

INTERPERSONAL EFFECTIVENESS

Innovative

Repairs	Many clients probably grew up, or are currently growing up, in families that didn't teach them how to make healthy repairs. Making repairs is about taking responsibility, apologizing when appropriate, accepting an apology when it makes sense, having the ability to let go and move on, and learning from the situation to avoid it in the future
Four Horsemen of the Apocalypse	This uses the metaphor of the Four Horsemen said to appear at the end of the world. If a client has the Four Horsemen in his or her relationships, then the relationship might be over. Criticism, contempt, defensiveness, and stonewalling may be the four most destructive behaviors in relationships.

The above Horsemen may not apply to these clients. Each client can identify their own Horsemen and then implement strategies to keep these destructive forces out of their relationships. Other Horsemen can be:

Youth	*Adults*
• Not communicating	• Dishonesty
• Withdrawal	• Not taking MH meds
• Dishonesty	• Out-of-control spending
• School refusal	• Credit card debt
• Playing video games	• Workaholism
• Bullying	• Drugs and alcohol
• Violence	• Violence
• Drugs & alcohol	• Infidelity
• Delinquency	• Internet sex/pornography

DBT SKILL ORIGINAL SOURCE

Mindfulness		Distress Tolerance		Emotional Regulation		Interpersonal Effectiveness	
Skill	Source	Skill	Source	Skill	Source	Skill	Source
Be Mindful	Marra, 2004	ACCEPTS	Linehan, 1993b	ABC	Linehan, 1993b	DEAR (WO)MAN	(Moonshine, 2007) Linehan 1993b
Body Scan	Moonshine, 2007	Crisis Survival Network	Moonshine, 2007	BEHAVIOR	Marra, 2004	Broken Record	Linehan, 1993b
Describe	Linehan, 1993b	Exploring Pros & Cons	Linehan, 1993b	Build Positive Emotions	Moonshine, 2007	Ignore	Linehan, 1993b
Effectively	Linehan, 1993b	Half Smile	Linehan, 1993b	CARES	Marra, 2004	Turn the Table	Linehan, 1993b
Mindful Eating	Moonshine, 2007	IMPROVE	Linehan, 1993b	EMOTIONS	Marra, 2004	GIVE	Linehan, 1993b
Moment to Pause	Moonshine, 2007	Keeping It In Perspective	Moonshine, 2007	Exploring Emotions	Marra, 2004	FAST	Linehan, 1993b
Non-Judgmental	Linehan, 1993b	OBJECTIVES	Marra, 2004	Feeling not Acting	Moonshine, 2007	Interactions in Relationships	Spradlin, 2003
Observe	Linehan, 1993b	Observe Breathing	Linehan, 1993b	Getting to Know Emotions	Marra, 2004	Relationship Thinking	Spradlin, 2003
ONE MIND	Marra, 2004	Radical Acceptance	Linehan, 1993b	Lemonade	Moonshine, 2007	Relationship Assumptions	Spradlin, 2003
One-Mindfully	Linehan, 1993b	Self Soothe	Linehan, 1993b	Love Dandelions	Moonshine, 2007	Rel. Mindfulness	Spradlin, 2003
Participate	Linehan, 1993b	Self Soothe First Aid Kit	Moonshine, 2007	MEDDSS	Linehan, 1993b	Dealing with Difficult People	Spradlin, 2003
Square Breathing	Moonshine, 2007	SPECIFIC PATHS	Marra, 2004	Opposite to Emotions	Linehan, 1993b	The Most Difficult	Spradlin, 2003
Turtling	Moonshine, 2007	Turning the Mind	Linehan, 1993b	Ride the Wave	Moonshine, 2007	Repairs	Spradlin, 2003
Wise Mind	Linehan, 1993b	Willingness	Linehan, 1993b	TRUST	Marra, 2004	4 Horsemen	Spradlin, 2003

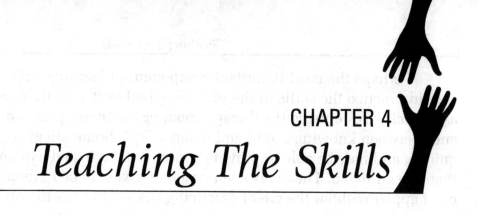

CHAPTER 4
Teaching The Skills

Many of the suggestions in this section will apply to teaching DBT skills, other skills, or other psychoeducational models. Learning needs to be accessible, relevant, engaging, fun, and interesting. Two major considerations of teaching skills are learning styles and attention span.

Learning Styles: Children, teenagers, and adults learn three ways: Auditorily, Visually, and Kinesthetically, and each person has a preferred style or way that he learns best. Some clients learn best by listening and talking about things. These clients are primarily auditory learners. Other clients will learn best through reading and visual representations. These clients are primarily visual learners. The last group includes clients whose optimal learning state happens through doing things, being active, and practicing things in their lives. These clients are kinesthetic learners. While each person has a preferred style or way they learn best, most clients can benefit from learning new concepts through a variety of styles.

When teaching DBT skills it is important to appeal to all three of these styles. Lecture or discussion about the skills is helpful and using visual representations of skills through media, posters, or objects is recommended.

Examples of auditory learning activities:

- Lecture
- Discussion
- Small-group exercises

Examples of visual learning activities:

- Written handouts
- PowerPoint presentations
- Art projects
- Games

Examples of kinesthetic learning activities:

- Art projects
- Games
- Role plays
- Small-group exercises

Perhaps the most important component of learning DBT is practice. Clients should practice the skills in the session, whether it is individual or group, as well as in their lives outside the therapy room or treatment program. There is a difference between knowing a skill and using a skill. Some clients can learn skills quickly and may be able to provide a more sophisticated explanation of the skill than the clinician. They may even coach or give advice to their peers. All of this can happen without the client practicing the skill in his life on a consistent basis.

An example of this occurred when a client enrolled in a treatment program with a significant DBT focus. This client enrolled in treatment because she was having problems with addiction, out-of-control relationships, and impaired parenting. The client had previously participated in a DBT group at another treatment center. She brought her old treatment binder to her first session of her new group. She did not participate during the group. At the end of the group she approached the group clinician and said she didn't think that she should have to participate in the group since she had been through DBT before. She pulled out her binder to prove that she had gone through DBT. Her reasoning was that it was similar to taking a college course: She had taken the group at another center, so she should receive credit for work already completed.

The group clinician listened to her reasoning and looked at the work she had completed. The group clinician asked questions about how she was using one or two skills as well as for examples of how the skills had been helpful with her recent troubles. The client was able to use the names of the skills and sometimes give accurate definitions but was unable to give a coherent example or demonstrate how she was using the skills. The clinician commented that she certainly had done some work in a previous group, thanked the client for sharing her treatment work, and then suggested that she could benefit from more practice and integration of the skills into her life. The client was somewhat unhappy with this response.

She then pleaded her case to her individual clinician. This clinician was aware of her request to the group clinician and took more time to process the request with the client. The client again was unable to give examples in sufficient detail to demonstrate the use of DBT skills in her daily life. The clinician validated the client's request and then explained that the continued difficulties in her life and her present unhappiness could probably be alleviated by her increased use of many of the skills. The clinician balanced the therapeutic dialectics of:

- Acceptance and Change
- Centeredness and Flexibility
- Nurturing and Benevolently Demanding

The clinician suggested that the client was using the skill of **Broken Record** by making multiple requests. The clinician then encouraged the client to use the skill of **Lemonade** instead, by refocusing her persistence and using her ability to ask for accommodations in ways that would serve her better and bring her more success. Through the therapeutic relationship and irreverent and supportive communication, the client was able to enter into a contract to stay in the group and to focus on actually using the skills in her life. Later in treatment the client commented that she had thought she knew the skills and was using them but she'd realized that she wasn't using them as much as she could. Upon making this realization she was able to discuss in significant detail different DBT skills and act out a number of the skills that she had found particularly helpful. She became an ally of the group clinician by encouraging other clients and pointing out discrepancies demonstrating that they might not be using the skills as much as they could be.

ATTENTION SPAN

While in some ways teenagers may have the capacity to pay attention longer than adults, both teenagers and adults have limited attention spans. Some clients have very long attention spans. Some activities can engage the attention span for an extended amount of time while other activities are only able to engage the attention span for a few minutes or seconds. When teaching the skills it is optimal to have a variety of activities. Don't do any one activity for too long. If the clinician is bored with an activity the clients may be bored as well. Activities to try:

- A little bit of lecture
- Video and music examples
- Handouts
- Small group activities
- Skits and charades
- Art work such as painting, modeling clay, or making collages
- Having the clients teach one another a skill
- Imagery and visualizations
- Role plays and in vivo practice
- Guest speakers

Observe and learn from the clients, and use what works for them. Learn from professional colleagues as well. Inquire how other clinicians teach skills, watch other clinicians work, or invite other clinicians to the group. DBT is hard work and having fun is a useful way to make it engaging and interesting.

Additional components to consider when teaching DBT skills include fostering motivation, tools that foster learning, and Cognitive-Behavioral interventions. Practice and homework assignments outside the individual or group therapy session are essential if clients are going to be successful in utilizing their DBT skills in real life situations.

MOTIVATIONAL STRATEGIES

Motivation is about what is in it for each person and part of the DBT focus is on balancing the dialectic of self-interest with investment in relationships with others. Self-interest in moderation, however, can be very effective. To build motivation to engage in DBT the clinician needs to find out what is important to the client: his values, goals, and who he wants to be. What is important to the client is an essential piece of building motivation. Each client has a variety of things that are important to him and may include the following:

Positive Frame	Negative Frame
• Being pain-free	• Having too much pain
• Emotional stability	• Emotionally out of control
• Clarity of thought	• Confusion
• Self-knowledge	• Feeling out of touch with oneself
• Being respected	• Being disrespected
• Being loved	• Being disliked, hated, or alone
• Loving others	• Disliking or hating others
• Functional family	• "Crazy" family
• Strong support system	• Problematic or no support system
• Financial independence	• Debt or dependence on others
• Stable, appropriate employment	• Under- or unemployment
• Stimulating career	• Directionless or passionless career
• Creative outlets	• Feeling unimaginative or uninspired
• Recreation and leisure	• Bored with nothing to do
• Ethics and morality	• No guiding principles
• Contributing to other's lives, local environment, or global community	• Isolation

Get to know what the client considers important and tailor the DBT skills and philosophy to assist him in having a sufficient amount of whatever he values. If he needs to increase one or more things that he considers important, choose skills that will help him to accomplish this. If the client believes he already has a good amount of what is important, focus on developing the skills to maintain those values.

Let's explore some of these. If a client wants to have more emotional stability, most of the emotional regulation skills are helpful. In particular the clinician might consider **Ride the Wave** and **TRUST**. If the client has established emotional stability and wants to maintain it, the clinician might suggest using **MEDDSS** daily and **Keeping It in Perspective** when indicated.

Another example would be in the area of clarity of thought. In the case of a client wanting to establish clarity of thought, the clinician might suggest **Wise Mind** or **OBJECTIVES**. When a client wants to maintain clarity of thought, focus on **Turning the Mind** and **Broken Record**.

Help the client to build a strong support system by teaching the skills of **Relationship Mindfulness** and **Interactions in Relationships**. To sustain healthy relationships the skills of **Repairs** and **Four Horsemen** are particularly useful.

Creative outlets, fun, and recreational opportunities can be increased by using the skills **Positive Emotional Experiences** and **ABC**. Maintaining creative outlets, fun, and recreational opportunities can be accomplished through the use of **Half-Smile** and **IMPROVES**.

One final example is ethics and morality. The skills of **Willingness** and **Radical Acceptance** would be useful to increase values. To maintain skills in the areas of ethics and morality, the client would benefit from using **BEHAVIOR** and **Turtling**.

These are just a few suggestions of skills. The clinician might choose different skills based on the situation, the unique aspects of the client, and the clinician's judgment.

Values are another important component to building motivation. A client may want to be a "good" person, parent, family member, student, employee, etc. Values might include doing the right thing, being the best person they can be, contributing through service work, volunteerism, and charity, as well as a connection with spiritual practices. By taking the client's values into consideration and weaving them into the clinical process, a clinician can help clients to build insight about how DBT's life perspective and determine which skills will work in their lives. Skills that support values include **Non-Judgmental**, **Wise Mind**, **Keeping It In Perspective**, and **BEHAVIOR**.

Most clients have a variety of goals they want to accomplish. When the clinician shows clients how they can use their skills to achieve their goals, they will see what is in it for them. Using the skill **Effectively** encourages clients to be efficient and intentional with their efforts. **Effectively** also helps clients keep their eye on the proverbial ball by avoiding distraction or undermining their own efforts. Other skills that are useful with accomplishing goals are **Lemonade**, **One-Mindfully**, **Turning the Mind**, and **FAST**.

Empowering clients to be who they want to be taps into their hope, optimism, and vision for the future, although it may be challenging to get clients to envision the future when they are in pain, engaging in unhealthy relationships or problematic or life-threatening behavior. One strategy is to start small. Help the client to achieve a small success and then build on it by using two Motivational Interviewing techniques: hypothetical change, and radical change (Miller & Rollnick, 2002).

Hypothetical change is a useful intervention for clients who can't imagine how their life could be any different. This intervention entails asking the client how someone in a similar situation in another time or place could change their life to be completely different. This might sound something like: "Hypothetically, let's say there is someone who looks a little like you and has a life similar to yours in a parallel universe. How would you assist this person to make the necessary changes in thinking, feeling, and behaving to reach their potential and be the person they want to be?" This engages clients in finding their own solutions and helps get them out of a typical hopeless perspective. There will also be a sense of pride in being able to provide advice and assistance to others, even if only hypothetically. Being hypothetical gives them the opportunity to think outside the box, suspend barriers and obstacles, and focus only on solutions.

The second strategy is radical change. Radical change is about envisioning that everything is different and any or all change is possible. A common therapeutic technique that illustrates radical change is the miracle question. This would sound something like "If you woke up tomorrow and all your problems were solved, what would your life look like?" or "Let's say that on your birthday (or January 1), you will be the person you want to be. Who would that person be?" This may be a technique you already use from your therapeutic tool kit.

When using either hypothetical or radical change, once the client has a vision about who they want to be or what they want their life to look like, the clinician and client work together to develop a plan to accomplish their vision. The plan needs to be both detailed and flexible. Help the client set himself up for success by setting small steps he can accomplish and normalize difficulties. One skill that is useful here is ***Keeping It In Perspective***. The skill of ***Lemonade*** lets clients take the skills they currently use to damage their lives or themselves and use them in an effective way to implement their vision. A client who tolerates considerable emotional or physical pain when harming himself can focus this ability to tolerate pain from working hard as well as on tolerating disappointments and setbacks.

Other Motivational Interviewing (MI) techniques are useful in building motivation for change and for integrating DBT philosophy and skills into daily life (Miller & Rollnick, 2002). MI charges the clinician to roll with the resistance that clients bring into the therapeutic process. Rolling with resistance includes eight interventions that can be divided into two categories: supportive and strategic. Supportive rolling with resistance interventions includes simple, amplified, and double-sided reflections. Reflection is repeating to a client what he has just communicated or has communicated in the past. Communication can be both verbal and nonverbal. Reflections can repeat the client's communication identically or nearly so. Clinicians can also rephrase or paraphrase client communication by using different words with very similar meanings. Reflecting back the client's emotions or feelings is a fourth way to use this type of interaction.

> *Simple Reflections* let the client know that the clinician understands him by reflecting back what the clinician hears or sees. An example of this would be:
>
> **Client:** "I don't see how this will help me."
> **Clinician:** "You can't imagine how this will make your life better."

Amplified Reflections are when a clinician adds emphasis or weight to a particular piece of the client's communication. For example:

Client: "I've tried stuff like this before and it never seems to work for long. I get really exhausted having to work so hard. I really wish my life was different. I wish I didn't have so many problems. It doesn't seem fair that others don't have it as hard as I do."

Clinician: "You've worked really hard. You've put a lot of effort into changing your life but it still remains the same."

Double-Sided Reflections explicitly acknowledge dialectics by bringing in both, or many, sides of how the client feels or thinks about something. Here is an example:

Client: "I really wish it wasn't so hard. I want my life to be better but I don't want to have to do all this work. Shouldn't I be better by now? When I started I was so hopeful that you could solve this for me and my life would be perfect."

Clinician: "So there is part of you that wants things to be better and another part of you that doesn't want to work so hard. You wish there was a way to change things and you had hoped that I could make everything all right."

Reflections affirm the client, illustrating that the clinician is paying attention and understands. They also foster the therapeutic relationship and validate the client. Once there is trust and a strong working relationship the clinician can utilize the strategic rolling with resistance techniques. These techniques include *Reframing, Agreement with a Twist, Shifting Focus, Emphasizing Personal Choice and Control,* and *Coming Alongside (Paradox).*

Reframing changes the meaning of what the client is talking about to help him see that change would be helpful.

Client: "I've tried a lot of things. I already know how to make things better."

Clinician: "So you have a lot of information and skills, we just need to figure out how to use them most effectively."

Agreement with a Twist is a reflection with a reframe. First the clinician reflects what the client is communicating and then reframes it.

Client: "There's no point. My life will never be better."

Clinician: "It feels like everything is hopeless and that things will never improve. I remember you telling me in the past that you didn't think your life would get better but then you really started to make changes. In the past you have taken hopelessness and turned it into energy and commitment to find a way to live life differently."

Shifting Focus is a useful intervention when the client feels overwhelmed, hopeless, or defensive. This entails changing the subject to a less intense or provocative subject, at least for a little while.

Client: "Why do we keep talking about this? This isn't helping me. What are you doing to help me? This feels like a complete waste of my time."

Clinician: "Maybe now isn't the time to talk about doing this differently. I remember at the beginning of the session you wanted to tell me about what a great weekend you had. Tell me more about that."

Emphasizing Personal Choice and Control puts the client in the driver's seat, much like the skill of Turning the Mind. Clients learn that it is up to them and that they have the ability to do it their way. This intervention is particularly useful for clients who feel forced to be in treatment as well as in cases where there is an explicit mandate.

Client: "I don't see why I have to be here. There's nothing you can tell me that will make a difference."

Clinician: "Being here seems pointless. It's really up to you to figure out how being here will be useful, what you want to learn, and how you might do things differently in your life."

Coming Alongside is a paradoxical intervention. Here the clinician predicts that the client cannot do it differently. This intervention is sometimes judged as manipulative and it doesn't work for some clinicians and certain clients. Passive, dependent clients probably won't get the most out of the technique but clients who are anti-authority, who need to be right, and who are contrary in nature often respond well to this intervention.

Client: "There's no point, I can't get it right. I'll never be successful. "

Clinician: "Staying the same seems to be the only option. You couldn't do it even if you really tried hard."

For more information on Motivational Interviewing see:

Motivational Interviewing, Second Edition: Preparing People for Change by William R. Miller and Stephen Rollnick, 2002.

Motivational Interviewing in the Treatment of Psychological Problems (Applications of Motivational Interviewing) by Hal Arkowitz, Hinny A. Westra, William R. Miller, and Stephen Rollnick, 2007.

A model related to Motivational Interviewing that is useful for increasing client's effective behavior is Stages of Change by Prochaska, Norcross, and DiClemente (1995). It is important to evaluate what stage of change (SOC) a client is in and use the accompanying interventions to facilitate forward movement. The stages include pre-contemplation, contemplation, preparation, action, maintenance, and relapse. Since change is a dynamic process it is most useful to consider the junctures between stages as the client moves from one stage to another.

The junctures are:

- Early Pre-contemplation
- Late Pre-contemplation → Early Contemplation
- Late Contemplation → Early Preparation
- Late Preparation → Early Action
- Late Action → Early Maintenance
- Late Maintenance → Relapse or return to old behavior

Early Pre-contemplation is characterized by clients thinking they don't have a problem. Interventions to facilitate forward movement support clients' strengths, explore goals, and raise awareness of problems and difficulties.

Suggested DBT skill: **Willingness**

Late Pre-contemplation → Early Contemplation is characterized by an emerging awareness of the problem and clients beginning to think about how to deal with it. Interventions that facilitate forward movement include normalizing that change is overwhelming at times, leveraging environmental and relational reasons for change, and tapping into previous successes.

Suggested DBT skill: **Pros and Cons**

Late Contemplation → Early Preparation is characterized by clients thinking about change and beginning to create a plan to make change happen. Interventions that facilitate forward movement include fostering intrapsychic reasons for change, tapping into clients' self-efficacy, and lowering obstacles to making a change.

Suggested DBT skill: **Lemonade**

Late Preparation → Early Action is characterized by continued plans to change and the beginning of behaviors to put change into place. Interventions that facilitate forward movement include announcing change plans, enlisting interpersonal support, and establishing success through small changes that come easily to the client.

Suggested DBT skill: **Participate**

Late Action → Early Maintenance is characterized by continued efforts to change and beginning to maintain changes that have been accomplished. Forward movement is facilitated by positively reinforcing the changes made, planning for challenging situations that provoke a return to old behaviors, and supporting the client's resolve to have a different life.

Suggested DBT skill: **SPECIFIC PATHS**

Early Maintenance → Late Maintenance is characterized by clients who maintain the changes they have made and adopting these changes into their daily life. Interventions here include illustrating self-efficacy, supporting effective problem-solving abilities, and normalizing bumps in the road.

Suggested DBT skill: ***Effectively***

Relapse or return to old behavior is returning to problematic behavior, re-engaging in self-injurious behavior, or returning to old systems. Sometimes clients actively engage in their relapse and sometimes relapse happens to them, particularly with mental health symptoms. Relapse can happen at any time during the change process. When a client is on the road to relapse, or has relapsed, the clinician can leverage the therapeutic relationship, evaluate factors leading to the relapse, and support the client's self-efficacy to reinstitute their DBT skills.

Suggested DBT skill: ***Turtling***

For more on Stages of Change, see:

Changing for Good: A Revolutionary Six-Stage Program for Overcoming Bad Habits and Moving Your Life Positively Forward by James O. Prochaska, John Norcross, and Carlo DiClemente (1995).

Motivational strategies address the fundamental question of why a client should be interested in learning DBT skills. If a client doesn't view learning certain information or skills as relevant to his needs or desires that client will not be motivated to invest the necessary effort in learning. Motivation to learn about DBT skills should never be assumed.

Developing client motivation to learn information and skills is critical for teaching each DBT module. Motivational strategies involve helping clients to see how learning information and skills will help them achieve short- and long-term goals. Some of the goals for DBT pertain to reduction of distress due to mental health symptoms, hopelessness, and destructive behaviors, while other goals may involve improving relationships, job or volunteer opportunities, recreational activities, or other desired changes.

Developing motivation for learning the information and skills contained in DBT is an ongoing and collaborative process that occurs throughout the treatment process. Motivation often needs to be rechecked or rekindled in the midst of teaching information or skills for which motivation may have previously been established. Motivation can wax and wane over time, especially if clients perceive their goals to be distant and difficult to achieve. To help clients sustain motivation clinicians need to convey their own confidence that the clients can achieve their goals and support clients' optimism, self-confidence, and self-efficacy.

VALIDATION AND COMMITMENT STRATEGIES

Validation and commitment strategies is yet another dialectic. Clinicians balance validating the client with gaining commitment to the treatment process. Clinicians need to provide enough of each of these while avoiding getting stuck in too much of either position.

Validation is done through supportive communication, reflective listening, cheerleading, and accepting the client's perception of reality. Validation lets clients know they are understood and appreciated for the individuals they are. Their experiences of reality are accepted as real for them even if the clinician or others might not experience things the same way. Validation creates safety and fosters the therapeutic relationship. Given that most clients have grown up in, and perhaps still live in, invalidating environments validation from a clinician can provide a corrective emotional experience. From the validation of the clinician clients can learn to validate and trust themselves. This can lead to increased confidence, empowerment, and self-efficacy.

Validation must, however, be balanced with commitment. DBT commitment strategies include **Playing Devil's Advocate**, **Foot in the Door**, **Door in the Face**, **Linking Present and Prior Commitments**, **Freedom to Choose**, and **Absence of Alternatives** (Linehan, 1993a; Linehan, 1993b; Miller, Rathus, & Linehan, 2006).

Playing Devil's Advocate: This is a paradoxical position where the clinician suggests the opposite position from what the client is saying. In the context of commitment, the clinician might say therapy is really hard and it might not be something the client wants to do. Since some clients have a contrary nature this strategy can encourage the client to argue for why they are investing in therapy and talk about how hard are they are going to work.

Foot in the Door: This strategy is based on the metaphor of the traveling salesman. Just get one foot in the door and then the clinician can find out what is important to the other person. In therapy, this is where the therapeutic relationship is fostered and little demand is made of the client for change.

Door in the Face: This is a strategic intervention that requires the clinician to push the client to do something really hard that they are likely to reject. Then the clinician asks for something easier instead. The client is more likely to commit to the second request for action because it seems less demanding. There may be a considerable amount of negotiation between the clinician and the client. Clients need see what is in it for them and figure out how they will integrate DBT into their lives.

Linking Present and Prior Commitments: This is a strength-based intervention that reviews how previous commitments to self and others have led to the client's sustaining effective change. Helping the client to realize that he has succeeded before makes it easier to continue with current commitments even when they are difficult or overwhelming.

Freedom to Choose: This is another strength-based intervention that shows the client that it's really up to him. He can choose what he wants to work on and how to work on it. There are limits to how a clinician might deal with a client. When a client wants to cut himself to express pain the clinician might not support this choice but can acknowledge the client's ability to make this choice. With choices come natural and logical consequences. A client's choice to continue to harming himself might result in limited access to the primary therapist. Thus the client's agenda is put on hold or he experiences negative reinforcement. As the client considers his freedom to choose and the accompanying natural and logical consequences, then he is able to make an informed decision about what is in his best interests.

Absence of Alternatives: This strategy utilizes the client's own hopelessness. If there are no other options, he might as well engage in this thing called DBT. Some clients are in so much pain that at least DBT can't make it worse. One question to ask would be: "How is that working for you?" If the client's current behavior isn't getting his needs met then maybe DBT can assist him in meeting needs more effectively and building a life worth living.

Clinicians should not only balance validation and commitment strategies but also be flexible in how they combine commitment strategies. For example, when using ***Devil's Advocate*** also use ***Previous Commitments***. When using ***Foot in the Door*** also use ***Door in the Face***. ***Absence of Alternatives*** balances nicely with ***Freedom to Choose***.

COGNITIVE-BEHAVIORAL STRATEGIES

Cognitive-behavioral strategies involve the systematic application of learning principles to help clients acquire and use DBT information and skills. A number of different cognitive-behavioral strategies are employed in helping clients master DBT skills.

REINFORCEMENT

Reinforcement can be broken down into two types: positive reinforcement and negative reinforcement. Positive reinforcement refers to an increase in something pleasant: a nice meal, money, a hug, praise, and working at an interesting job. Negative reinforcement refers to a decrease in something pleasant, or an increase in something unpleasant. Examples of negative reinforcement include increased feelings of anxiety, anger, or being hung-over, and increased rates of relapse or hospitalization. Negative reinforcement should not be confused with punishment, which is something unpleasant that is intentionally imposed by an external authority in response to behavior.

The principles of reinforcement play an important role in teaching DBT because its core goals are by their very nature reinforcing. Positive reinforcement occurs when the client experiences success, empowerment, improvement in relationships, and increased life satisfaction. Negative reinforcement occurs when the client has more difficulties, discomfort, and pain that cannot be removed. As clients learn and apply the skills taught in DBT they will accomplish some of their goals and live consistently with their values. As they have more and more experience of having the life they want to have and being the person they want to be, using the skills is positively reinforced which encourages increased use of the skills.

The clinician uses positive social reinforcement in the form of cheerleading and encouragement so that clients learn the skills and experience success when using them. This type of social reinforcement is important because it acknowledges the client's efforts and makes the client feel good about himself.

As clients learn to use the skills for managing their symptoms and making progress towards recovery, they experience the naturally reinforcing effects of these skills, including reductions in distress, increases in self-sufficiency, and attainment of their goals. Clinicians need to work closely with clients and monitor progress toward goals to ensure that these positive outcomes of DBT are attained.

SHAPING

Shaping refers to reinforcement of successive approximations to a goal. The expression "Rome wasn't built in a day" summarizes the concept of shaping. Similar to the building of Rome, the information and skills taught in DBT take time to learn, with each client learning at his own pace. Practicing complex skills, such as Non-judgmental, Radical Acceptance, and Opposite to Emotions, and the acronyms can truly help clients to understand and integrate these skills into their lives. It is important for the clinician to recognize the steps taken along the way and to provide ample positive feedback and encouragement.

Even when the pace of learning is quite slow and each step forward is small, clinicians can acknowledge these gains by pointing them out, praising efforts, and letting clients know they are making progress. Taking a "shaping attitude" means that clinicians understand the amount of time and effort required to learn the information and skills in DBT and provide frequent reinforcement to clients as they progress.

MODELING

One of the most powerful methods for teaching someone a skill is to demonstrate it. Modeling refers to the demonstration of skills for the purposes of teaching. Modeling has an important role to play in teaching DBT, especially in helping clients learn new skills. When modeling a new skill it is useful for the clinician to first describe the nature of the skill and then to explain that the skill will be demonstrated to show how it works. The clinician then models the skill and, when completed, obtains feedback from the client about what he observed and how effective the skill appeared to be.

The clinician can tell a story about how he used the skill in his life without disclosing too much personal information or the clinician can tell a story about how someone he knew used a skill. The clinician can ask the clients if they know anyone who appears to use the skill that is being taught. Another illustration would be the clinician acting out how he imagines the client would use the skill and demonstrating it in the session. Modeling the skill in a variety of ways can give the client concrete examples of how to use the skills and the benefits the skills could provide. This can be a very useful step in the client successfully using skills that are being taught.

BEHAVIORAL TAILORING

Behavioral tailoring involves helping clients to develop strategies that incorporate skills and behaviors that will serve them well into their daily lives. As the client learns the DBT skills, she can work with the clinician to determine the skills most useful to him. The client and clinician can develop a plan to integrate these skills into the client's day-to-day experiences.

The rationale behind behavioral tailoring is that building the application of skills and desired behaviors into an existing routine will provide clients with regular cues to use their skills thereby minimizing the chances that they will forget. Interest in using skills, or in applying a desired behavior, can be established by motivational techniques including eliciting and reviewing the advantages (e.g., reduced symptoms, relapses, and re-hospitalizations) and making progress toward client goals. Diary cards are also useful with behavioral tailoring; see the homework section below for further explanation.

When using behavioral tailoring, the clinician first explores the client's daily routine, including activities such as self-care, activities of daily living, work, family relationships, and recreational pursuits. Then clinician and client then identify an activity that can be adapted to include the application of DBT skills. In order to ensure that this plan is carried out the clinician may first model the routine for the client and then engage the client in a role-play of the same routine. After rehearsing the routine in session, the clinician and the client could establish a homework assignment to implement the plan. Successful implementation of the behavioral tailoring plan could be reinforced by praising the client for following through.

PRACTICE AND ROLE PLAY

The expression "practice makes perfect" is well-suited to learning DBT. In order to be learned, DBT skills need to be practiced both inside and outside of sessions. Practice helps clients become more familiar with a DBT skill, identifies obstacles to using the skill outside of sessions, and provides opportunities for feedback from the clinician and others. It is only by practicing skills outside of the sessions that clients can improve their ability to manage their symptoms, reach optimal functioning, and increase life satisfaction.

Practice of DBT skills in session is especially effective when it is combined with modeling by the clinician although it may be done without such modeling. One of the best methods to help clients practice a DBT skill is for the clinician to set up a role-play that will allow the client to use the skill in the kind of situation that may come up in his life. After a skill has been practiced the clinician should always note some strengths of the client's performance and strive to be as specific as possible. The clinician may also choose to give some suggestions to the client about how the skill may be done even more effectively and additional practice in the session may be helpful.

HOMEWORK ASSIGNMENTS

Practicing DBT skills as a homework assignment between sessions is an essential part of DBT. There is a difference between knowing skills and using them. Clients may be able to learn the skills, and even demonstrate the skills in session, but if they don't use the skills outside of therapy or treatment they are going to get very little out of them. For this reason clinicians must assign practice homework.

One homework assignment that requires the client to demonstrate the use of DBT skills is keeping diary cards. Diary cards ask the client to track their use of the skill. In the beginning of this process the clinician asks the client to record the number of times he uses a skill. This can be a tally in the client's day planner (either paper or electronic), check marks in his checkbook register, on his mp3 player—whatever works for the client. It is human nature to do more of something when we are counting it and wanting to increase it. The reverse also works when trying to decrease or reduce something. An example of reducing something is the "swear jar." If children are using profanity or "swear words" their parents can start a "swear jar" that requires the children to pay each time they swear. Their increased awareness and the actual cost of swearing will help children to significantly reduce their swearing. The same principle applies to using DBT skills. The more the client tracks use of the skills and behaviors to be reduced or eliminated, the more often the skills will be used and the less often unhelpful or harmful behaviors will be used.

Diary cards are also useful to the clinician. It shows what skill the client is using and how often. If there are difficulties using the skills the clinician can work with the client to reduce or eliminate the difficulties. When the client uses the skills and documents that on the diary cards the clinician can positively reinforce the skills and hear success stories.

Clients will commonly forget to complete their diary cards at first. It is important to continue to hold the expectation of completing the cards. If the clinician lets the client "off the hook" for keeping the cards the client will get less out of DBT and run the risk of not implementing the skills in their lives at all.

Not practicing the skills between sessions and failing to complete diary cards are considered major therapy-interfering behaviors (See Chapter 1). Clinicians need to acknowledge these therapy-interfering behaviors, address the issues, hold the client accountable, and reinforce maintaining the diary cards by limiting the focus on the client's agenda until there is adequate investment in practicing skills and completing the cards. If the clinician fails to hold the client responsible and invests in the client's agenda, only reinforces that the skills and diary cards aren't important. It is essential to avoid this message.

RELAPSE PREVENTION

Relapse can be defined as a return of symptoms or difficulties, re-engaging in self-destructive behavior, or using alcohol or other drugs (AOD). Sometimes clients actively participate in their relapses by not taking medications, reducing self-care efforts, reengaging in problematic relationships, reengaging in self-harming behavior, or using AOD. At other times relapses occur for reasons out of the client's control such as the cyclical nature of bipolar and seasonal affective disorders. Relapses can also be brought on by environmental stressors such as losing a job or income source, family member illness, cars breaking down, or losing housing. Recovery, in this context, means that clients are living optimally, at their highest level of functioning and life satisfaction. Recovery can include being substance-free but not necessarily if the client is not addicted to substances. Recovery means living beyond symptoms and diagnoses to be the best person a client can be.

Relapse prevention is about helping the client identify warning signs of returning to old problematic behaviors or being at risk of using substances again. The client enlists a support system to assist him in watching for warning signs. When a warning sign has been identified the client can utilize a variety of DBT skills, receive support from family and friends, attend community support meetings, or talk with their clinician. By identifying and dealing with warning signs clients can avoid or minimize a relapse to their problematic behavior or substance use. Even if the client relapses to their old behavior or begins to use substances it is still better to catch it in progress so that the client can intervene quickly and effectively before the relapse is full-blown. Developing effective relapse prevention plans requires knowledge of and success with DBT skills.

When developing relapse prevention plans the clinician guides clients through a discussion of what a relapse might look like, what brings it on, and how to avoid a relapse. As part of this process, it will probably be useful to review previous relapses and highlight any client insights or clinician observations that will minimize future relapses. An informal relapse prevention plan could be:

Warning Sign: _____

DBT Skill: _____

Outcome: _____

If warning sign continues or worsens, contact support system or a helping professional.

RECOVERY PLANNING

A strength-based parallel to relapse prevention planning is recovery planning. Since DBT is designed to empower clients to build a life worth living it makes sense that most clinicians would develop a recovery plan with their clients. One suggested plan is:

RECOVERY PLAN

Recovery is about being the best possible person. It is about reaching your potential while dealing with difficulties, stress, and problems. Recovery is about effectively dealing with mental health and substance use problems. It also entails effectively dealing with family and support systems, jobs, meaningful activities, recreational opportunities, and having fun, just to name a few. The next few pages provide an opportunity to develop a recovery plan which can then be implemented.

This is my plan for recovery and optimal functioning:

> Which DBT Skills are most helpful for me?

> _____

> _____

> _____

1. **Practicing MEDDSS daily establishes a healthy self-care regimen.**

   a. Exercise

   _____

   _____

   b. Diet: Balanced and nutritious

   _____

   _____

   c. Drugs: Prescribed medication as directed and don't use illicit drugs

   _____

   _____

   d. Sleeping: A healthy amount

   _____

   _____

2. Prevention of Relapse or Return to Old Problematic Behavior:

a. The most important warning signs of problems reoccurring:

_____

_____

b. When I notice the warning signs, I will use the following DBT Skills:

_____

_____

3. Healthy Support System:

These are the people in my support system that support my recovery and use of DBT skills:

_____

_____

4. Having Fun and Recreation is an important part of recovery:

a. I will ensure that I have time for fun and recreation in my life on a regular basis by using the following strategies:

_____

_____

b. These are the fun and recreational activities that I will participate in on a regular basis that support my recovery:

_____

_____

c. I will utilize community support meetings by:

_____

_____

5. Dealing with Stress:

a. The most stressful things in my life are:

_____

_____

b. What DBT skills will I use to manage my stress?

_____

_____

6. Recovery Goals:

a. What progress have I made toward my recovery?

_____

_____

b. What am I currently working on in my recovery?

_____

_____

c. What will I do to maintain positive changes and continue my growth?

_____

_____

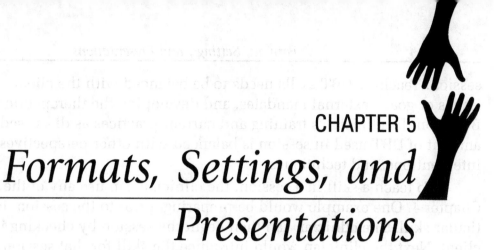

CHAPTER 5

Formats, Settings, and Presentations

FORMATS

DBT can be delivered in a variety of formats including individual therapy sessions, group therapy sessions, case management appointments, medication management outreach visits, recreation activities, or by spending unstructured time in the therapeutic community, classroom, or at home with family and friends.

DBT can be practiced as an exclusive modality, a primary model with a few other models, in an integrated manner along with multiple other modalities, or on an as-needed basis by using just a few components or skills. Determining how much DBT is woven into the clinical process should be based on education and training in DBT, DBT clinical supervision, the extent to which the theory resonates with the clinician, the types of clients treated, and the problems and symptoms of individual clients.

Setting also has an impact on the amount of DBT used in the clinical process. Private practice clinicians may have the flexibility to choose their therapeutic modalities and interventions but this may also be influenced by who is paying for treatment: an insurance company, employer, school, family, or the client. Private practice clinicians are also accountable to the client who either explicitly requests a specific therapy, such as DBT, or who presents with particular symptoms, such as self-harming behavior. Clinicians working at a treatment program or facility typically need to provide treatment consistent with regulations, as well as facility philosophy and policies. With its many components, DBT is a model that can be adapted and reorganized to work in a variety of ways.

INDIVIDUAL SESSIONS

Teaching clients the DBT philosophy and skills can be an integral part of meetings with their individual clinicians. In individual sessions motivation and learning can be tailored specifically to each client. The client's history and information from previous sessions can be used as examples of when a client has already used a skill or how a skill could be helpful. Metaphors can be applied specifically to the individual client's life.

When using DBT in individual sessions, skills teaching should only be a portion of what is covered. Depending on the client, the issues being addressed, and the client's informed consent, DBT skills may be 10–75% of what happens in session. Teaching DBT skills needs to be balanced with the client's agenda, new issues or goals, external mandates, and developing the therapeutic relationship. Based on the clinician's training and current practices as discussed above, the amount of DBT used in session is balanced with other perspectives, modalities, interventions, and techniques.

To teach a skill in a session, the clinician can use any of the suggestions in Chapter 4. One example would be preparing, prior to the session, to teach a particular skill. The clinician can then begin the session by checking in with the client. Next the clinician would introduce the skill for that session. The clinician would define the skill. The client might think about how she has used the skill or has known people who have used the skill even if they didn't know its name or why it was useful. Next there might be a role-play opportunity or visualization of how the client could use the skill in his life.

Wrapping up the educational process would include a short exploration of potential barriers along with ways to problem-solve these obstacles. Part of dealing effectively with barriers and obstacles is using the DBT skills even when there is no immediate solution to a problem. It is important for clients to know that using any set of skills will be challenging and imperfect. If they think it is easy and that the skills will always work perfectly, they are at risk for giving up early when they discover that it takes effort and doesn't always work. At the completion of the barriers and obstacles conversation, the clinician requests that the client use the skill as much as possible from then until the next session. This is where the clinician would request use of the diary card.

The rest of the session could be spent on other things the clinician has on his agenda or the client can be in the driver's seat with the direction of the session. When a skill is taught at the beginning of the session the client typically will make reference to the skill later in the session when he is talking about what is important to him. As the client is reflecting on his life, the client might see that the skill might work well for them. The client might also remember times that he already did something similar to the skill. Because the client and clinician will find ways to reference the skill taught earlier in the session it is preferable to teach the skill at the beginning of the session for 5-20 minutes. If the skill is taught at the end of session this opportunity is missed and time might run out before the skill can be fully explored.

Another example of how DBT skills can be integrated into individual sessions is to spontaneously teach a skill based on the issues the client is currently processing. This would happen when the clinician is listening to the client and realizes that a particular skill would be useful in this situation. At that point the clinician can dive into teaching the skill if he feels comfortable; he can get out any reference material or handouts to discuss the skill with the client; or he can make a note and prepare to teach the skill in the next session. Once the skill has been chosen the clinician will probably use a process similar to the one explained above.

A third method includes developing single or multiple treatment plans with DBT skills as the planned interventions. Here the client's presenting problem is identified, the treatment goal is determined, and then an appropriate skill can be chosen to meet the goal. The clinician then plans the method of teaching the skill, decides on practice opportunities, and selects homework assignments. Dialectics are typical items on treatment plans. Some examples might include "Independence and Investment in Relationships with Others," "Increase Self-Efficacy while Accepting Deficiencies," "Take Medication for Mental Health Problem while Learning Skills," or "Improve Physical Health and Accept Body Image."

GROUP THERAPY

DBT can be used at least two ways in group. The first is by having a curriculum and a lesson plan for each group. A group curriculum can either include a focus on all four modules or it can be dedicated to a particular module such as a mindfulness group or an emotional regulation group. A group can also offer skills from all four modules devoting several weeks to the same module. For example:

> Month 1: Mindfulness Skills
>
> Month 2: Emotional Regulation Skills
>
> Month 3: Distress Tolerance Skills
>
> Month 4: Interpersonal Effectiveness Skills

Another option would be to take a different week of the month for a skill from each module:

> Week 1: Mindfulness Skills
>
> Week 2: Emotional Regulation Skills
>
> Week 3: Distress Tolerance Skills
>
> Week 4: Interpersonal Effectiveness Skills

When an entire group or individual session is focused on a DBT skill, the preferred structure is:

First Third of the Session:

- Review homework
- Have client(s) display how the skill was used
- Practice skill if the client(s) didn't do the homework

Second Third of the Session:

- Introduce the new skill
- Teach the skill with creativity, interaction, and in a manner that appeals all three learning styles
- Give examples of how to use the skill
- Ask clients if they have had experience with the skill or something similar

Last Third of the Session:

- Practice or role-play the skill
- Discuss barriers and obstacles and how to effectively overcome them
- Assign the skill to be practiced between now and the next session

Here is how a four-month curriculum could be organized:

Month 1	Week 1: Mindfulness	*Wise Mind*
	Week 2: Distress Tolerance	*Crisis Survival Network*
	Week 3: Emotional Regulation	*Ride the Emotion*
	Week 4: Interpersonal Effectiveness	*Making Repairs*
Month 2	Week 1: Mindfulness	*Observe/Describe/Participate*
	Week 2: Distress Tolerance	*Self-Soothe and S.S. 1st Aid Kit*
	Week 3: Emotional Regulation	*Opposite to Emotion*
	Week 4: Interpersonal Effectiveness	*Four Horsemen*
Month 3	Week 1: Mindfulness	*Turtling*
	Week 2: Distress Tolerance	*Radical Acceptance*
	Week 3: Emotional Regulation	*TRUST*
	Week 4: Interpersonal Effectiveness	*GIVE and FAST*
Month 4	Week 1: Mindfulness	*Non-Judgmentally*
	Week 2: Distress Tolerance	*Half-Smile*
	Week 3: Emotional Regulation	*MEDDSS*
	Week 4: Interpersonal Effectiveness	*DEAR WOMAN or MAN*

The second way of teaching skills in group would be spontaneously. Here the clinician could pick a skill based on the content of what the clients bring in for group that session. This would be similar to the spontaneous option under "Individual Session" discussed above. This method takes considerable knowledge of DBT and confidence on the part of the clinician.

CASE MANAGEMENT APPOINTMENTS

These appointments are typically focused on meeting basic needs, connecting with community resources, and advocacy. DBT skills can be taught to clients to help them meet their own needs and to deal with frustration, setbacks, and other difficulties. DBT skills can empower clients to be effective in asking for help, getting needs met, maintaining housing, investing in healthy relationships, and engaging in meaningful activities such as employment or service work. Case managers, social workers, and other staff can introduce a skill, build motivation, practice the skill with the client, and encourage the client to use the skill in his life.

MEDICATION MANAGEMENT

Psychiatric prescribers and primary care physicians can teach and reinforce the use of DBT skills in addition to providing medication management. In particular **MEDDSS** is a fairly straightforward skill and is directly applicable to medical appointments. This can be done in collaboration with other clinicians or treatment teams or it can be done independently if the client doesn't have additional contact with mental health staff.

OUTREACH VISITS

Working with clients in their own environments is a great opportunity to facilitate their adoption of skills in their lives. Outreach clinicians can see the client's strengths and challenges firsthand; they can then choose the most appropriate skills and teach them in vivo and clients can ask for help as they run into difficulties. Seeing how the client makes use of the idea of balance and implements the skills allows multiple opportunities for positive reinforcement.

An example would be using **ACCEPTS** when a client is very upset about not getting what he wants. An outreach worker can teach the skill of **Wise Mind** when the client is out of balance with thinking or feeling. The skill of **Willingness** is useful when things are going badly for a client.

RECREATION ACTIVITIES

Skills can be woven into games, arts and crafts, listening to music, and sports. See Chapter 6 for "D.B.T. in Life™" games that include a board game, playing cards Bingo, and the Bonanza Dice Game. Staff or family members can teach clients skills and reinforce their use during these activities. Particularly when working with teenagers, the clinician can access multiple media to reinforce learning. This can include video games, music, music videos, movies, and the Internet. Having fun learning DBT skills makes it more likely that clients will use the skills in a variety of situations in their lives.

Clients can look for examples of skills being used in TV shows or in songs. For example the song "Sweet Escape" by Gwen Stefani and Akon illustrates **DEAR WOMAN**. "Big Girls Don't Cry" by Fergie illustrates **FAST**. **Radical Acceptance** is embedded in "Not Ready to Make Nice" by the Dixie Chicks. Another way to use TV or movies is to pick a difficulty or a conflict that a character is experiencing and have the clients decide what skills would be useful for the character and why.

When playing sports clients are often trying to be as **Effective** as possible. Not doing as well as desired, or losing, is an opportunity to use **Ride the Wave** or **Love Dandelions**.

Arts and crafts are ways that clients can create graphic illustrations of skills. Drawing the path they're on and all the twists and turns their path has taken is one way that clients can show how they use **Turning the Mind**. **Ride the Wave**, **Lemonade**, and **Turtling** can also easily be turned into a craft project.

UNSTRUCTURED TIME IN THE THERAPEUTIC COMMUNITY

This is one of the best opportunities to coach clients use of skills, as well as providing many opportunities to reinforce skills. All staff and clients can learn the skills as they help one another use them. It is this type of ongoing practice opportunity that will ensure clients' success when they return to their own environment fulltime.

Some of the examples from Recreational Activities can also be used here. Staff and other clients can comment when they see a client using a skill such as **DEAR MAN**, **Non-Judgmental**, or **Self-Soothe 1st Aid** Kit. Asking the question "How can you use your skills?" reminds the clients about their skills and gently holds them accountable for using them. This is an appropriate intervention for nearly all staff to use.

IN THE CLASSROOM

Skills can be woven into lesson plans. Teachers and school counselors can focus on teaching skills that will resonate with specific age groups and they can teach them in developmentally appropriate language. Using play therapy and expressive therapies reinforces learning for children and teenagers. Lots of repetition goes a long way toward ensuring that learning happens and that it will be transferred to home life. It is also very useful to orient family members to the skills (see below).

In addition to the suggestions in Recreational Activities and Unstructured Time, skills can be illustrated in stories. For example, "The Old Man and The Sea" by Ernest Hemingway contains several skills including **Feeling not Acting**, **Keeping It in Perspective**, and **Half-Smile**. Moments in history show the use of skills. For example the Industrial Revolution illustrates **Effectively** and **SPECIFIC PATHS**. Alexander Graham Bell used **Crisis Survival Network** when he called out for his assistant while inventing the telephone. There are many more examples that teachers can find nearly every day in their professional duties.

AT HOME WITH FAMILY AND FRIENDS

When a client's family and friends learn DBT skills it gives the client's family and friends the opportunity to apply the skills in their own lives and appreciate the complexities of them. In addition their familiarity with the skills provides opportunities for coaching and positive reinforcement. Family and friends can ask the same questions as clinical staff, such as "How did your skills help with this?" They can then give feedback if there is an opportunity to use the skill more effectively or say "good job" when it is used well.

When a client is having difficulty remembering to use **Non-Judgmental** with himself or with others, family and friends can gently remind the client and can help the client overcome any barriers. Friends and family can practice **Square Breathing**, **Pros and Cons**, **Opposite to Emotions**, or **Turn the Tables** with the client as well.

SETTINGS

DBT has been used in a variety of settings across the country, including private practice, outpatient group practice or agency, intensive outpatient or day treatment as well as in residential or inpatient programs. DBT can be used with success in these settings when treating mental health, addictions, and co-occurring disorders.

Private practice:

- Don't be the client's only resource
- Balance skills with client focus
- Emphasize usefulness of skills to client needs
- Assign homework and review regularly
- Consider joining a consultation group

Outpatient group practice or agency:

- Orient all team members to DBT
- Have two or more clinicians implement the model
- Connect the model with treatment philosophy and existing clinical practices
- Set up implementation for success
- Teach and review DBT in both individual and group sessions

Intensive outpatient or day treatment:

- Train staff on the basics of DBT and have them use their skills at work
- Create diary cards that are specific to the program
- Reinforce learning in the milieu at every opportunity
- Coach and give feedback regularly
- Tie most or all clinical services to DBT
- Use repetition and demonstration

Residential and inpatient programs:

- All staff play an essential role
- Milieu and support staff can coach and reinforce skills
- Use expressive therapies
- Weave DBT skills and philosophy into treatment philosophy
- Have staff demonstrate skills
- Have staff use skills to foster resilience in the workplace

Adapting for diversity:

Pamela Hays (2007) created an acronym for considering clients' diversity variables:

A = Age

D = Developmental strengths and weaknesses

D = Disabilities, both congenital and acquired

R = Religion and spirituality

E = Ethnicity

S = Socio-economical status

S = Sexual orientation

I = Indigenous heritage and First Peoples

N = National legacy

G = Gender identity, role and expression

AGE

Clients can be divided into four age groups: Children, teenagers/young adults, adults, and older adults.

Children are considered age 13 years and younger. Clinicians should select only a few skills with this age group such as *Turtling*, *Lemonade*, *Ride the Wave*, and the *Four Horsemen;* this group includes one skill from each of the four modules. These skills can be taught with developmentally appropriate language and visual images and toys can be used to illustrate the skills. When teaching skills to children use simple language and use the skills in a variety of ways. Utilize play therapy techniques, lots of repetition, and include the family in the reinforcement process.

Teenage Mutant Ninja Turtle videos, comics, and action figures can be used when teaching *Turtling*. The Teenage Mutant Ninja Turtles use cool language, skateboard, and eat pizza—things children love to do. The Teenage Mutant Ninja Turtles also display teamwork and collaboration and they work for the greater good—all while having fun. *Lemonade* can be taught by making lemonade, planting, growing, or visiting a lemon tree, or drawing lemons. Using artwork, visualization, and videos of surfing are ways to reinforce learning the skill of *Ride the Wave*. The *Four Horsemen* skill is about the destructive factors in relationships. For children their "horses" might be excessive energy, disobeying parents, disruptive behavior, eating sugar, incontinence, bullying or being combative, or not eating. Children can learn that when their horses are out of control it gets them into trouble and important adults are unhappy with them. Children can have toy horses and learn to control their horses so that they are well behaved while having fun.

Teenagers and young adults tend to range from 13 to 25 years old. There is a wide range of cognitive and emotional abilities in this age range. Choose skills that will appeal to their strengths and teach them in fun and interesting ways. Use multimedia to illustrate skills and to provide practice opportunities. Be sure to have them demonstrate their use of skills because it is possible for clients to know the skills intellectually without putting them into action in their lives. Suggested skills for teenagers and young adults are **Turning the Mind**, **Willingness**, **Self-Soothe 1st Aid Kit**, **Non-Judgmental**, **MEDDSS**, and **Wise Mind**.

Adults can range from mid-20s to mid-60s. It is important to choose skills that are relevant to adult clients and that foster motivation and empower self-efficacy. Evaluate where the adults are out of balance then strategize ways to create more balance. Build motivation by tapping into self-interest, values, and goals. Develop awareness of what skills a client is already using without knowing they are DBT skills. Suggested skills are **Effectively**, **Crisis Survival Network**, **ABC**, and **DEAR WOMAN or MAN**.

The last age group is older adults. Depending on which source you consult, this age group starts around age 55 to 68 years-old. People are living longer and may be very active in their senior years. In the 100 years between 1900 and 2000 life expectancy in the U.S. increased by nearly 25 years. Some older adults are living with chronic diseases whose effects must be factored into treatment. When teaching DBT skills also take into account the client's own life course as well as historical events that the client has lived through and adapt to the client's cognitive abilities. Suggested skills are **Participate**, **Radical Acceptance**, **Love Dandelions**, and **Repairs**.

DEVELOPMENTAL STRENGTHS AND WEAKNESSES

To assess this area clinicians will want to determine whether the client's developmental process has been within normal limits. In what ways did the client develop more quickly or slowly than the prototype of the typical developmental process? Evaluate the client's deficits and strengths and consider the impact of any abuse, trauma, or loss that may be present. Teach skills that support empowerment and resiliency. Developmental variables and age go hand-in-hand. Excelling developmentally can propel clients toward being more at home in the next older age group. Problematic or impaired development can lead to clients being members of a younger age group. Take all of this into account when choosing skills such as **Effectively**.

DISABILITIES

Consider the impact of disabilities and abilities. These can be physical, cognitive, developmental, emotional, or psychological so be sure to screen for both visible and invisible disabilities. Choose skills that foster independence and resiliency such as **Lemonade**, **MEDDSS**, **Non-Judgmental**, **GIVE**, and **FAST**.

RELIGION AND SPIRITUALITY

Be supportive and inclusive if the client has a religious or spiritual practice in their life and minimize the impact of shame and guilt if present. Match values and beliefs with skills such as **Turtling**. Turtles carry the world on their back in the Hindu religion and from this religion's perspective they have an extremely important role in maintaining balance. Tap into a community's support opportunities if that is useful for the client. Suggested skills are ***Turtling*** and ***OBJECTIVES***.

ETHNICITY

This may focus on physical attributes such as skin color. Many communities of color have a culture that is unique to that group. This includes African and Black, Latino, Asian, and Caucasian heritages. A "White" culture also exists, despite common belief to the contrary. Culture includes shared beliefs, rituals, holidays, values, and relationships. When working with a variety of ethnic groups temper curiosity with respect. Learn from the clients and do any needed homework outside of the clinical process.

Be inclusive of values and worldviews. Don't underestimate either current or historical impact of racism, discrimination, and oppression. Be sure to consider the ethnic community's perspective on mental health and substance use problems and the role of counseling. Some ethnic communities are supportive of counseling while in other groups it is highly stigmatized. Suggested skills are ***Self-Soothe 1st Aid Kit*** and ***Dealing with Difficult People***.

SOCIO-ECONOMIC STATUS

This variable concerns money, lifestyle, social status, and education. Consider the impact of poverty and privilege. Where indicated help the client access resources to meet his basic needs. Evaluate lifestyle strengths and weaknesses and empower clients to use skills to live more effectively. Consider how this category interacts with all the other diversity components. Suggested skills are ***Non-Judgmental*** and ***Keeping it in Perspective***.

SEXUAL ORIENTATION

This variable considers whom individuals are emotionally, physically, and psychologically attracted to. This includes heterosexuality, which means that attraction occurs between people of opposite sexes. The acronym LGTBQQI summarizes other possible orientations.

- L = Lesbians are women who are attracted to and have relationships with other women.
- G = Gays are men who are attracted to and have relationships with other men.
- T = Transgendered individuals are psychologically the opposite sex from their physical sex.
- B = Bisexual individuals are attracted to, and have relationships with, both women and men.
- Q = Queers are any non-heterosexual individuals.
- Q = Questioning individuals aren't sure of their sexual orientation.
- I = Intersex individuals have part or all of both sets of sex organs.

When working with LGTBQQI clients assess for internalized homophobia and psychological distress related to sexual orientation. Assist with the "coming out" process where indicated. Connect clients who are members of a particular group with allies and community supports that are present in many major cities and on the Internet. Suggested skills are **Crisis Survival Networks** and **Dealing with the Most Difficult**.

INDIGENOUS HERITAGE AND FIRST PEOPLES

This group includes Americans Indians, Alaskan Indians, and any group that is indigenous to an area. With this group be sure to integrate their values, world-view, perspective on health and healing, any connections to nature, and the importance of their ancestors. When selecting skills based on this information a clinician might choose **Turtling** because turtles are very important symbols to some American Indian and First Peoples communities. This diversity component tends to interact with religion, ethnicity, and socio-economic status. Suggested skills are **Turtling** and **Half-Smile**.

NATIONAL LEGACY

This variable may have a current impact on clients who are immigrants or are their family's first generation in this county. It may be more of a historical context for clients from families that immigrated during previous generations but clinicians should consider both current and historical factors. Pay attention to trauma that occurred in the home country even if it didn't happen directly to the client. For example a client of German heritage and Jewish descent may be affected by the Holocaust even though he wasn't there because his family members were imprisoned. Foster pride and tradition as long as they don't lead to judgments against other groups. Evaluate discrepancies with the dominant culture for any stress that this may cause. Suggested skills are **Wise Mind** and **Build Positive Emotions**.

GENDER IDENTITY, ROLE, AND EXPRESSION

Identity is the meaning that being a man or woman has for the client. Role refers to the typical expectations, activities, and duties of men and women for this client and in the community in which the client lives. Expression is about how the client chooses to live as a man or a woman, including the client's concepts of masculinity and femininity. This category is quite dynamic with other diversity components. When teaching DBT skills be sure to adapt metaphors and skills to the gender identity, role, and expression each individual client has. Suggested skills are **DEAR WOMAN or MAN**, **GIVE**, and **FAST**.

PITFALLS

Below is a list of potential pitfalls that clinicians should consider. Clinicians can develop strategies to minimize or avoid these pitfalls and other bumps in the road.

- Too many skills
- Going too fast
- Using it "right off the shelf"
- Not checking on homework
- Not having clients demonstrate skills
- Not using diary cards

- Ineffective self-care of the clinician
- Clinicians not using DBT skills themselves
- Countertransference challenges
- Falling into Anti-DBT Tactics (See Chapter 1).

CLINICAL PRESENTATIONS

- Anger
- Anxiety
- Bipolar
- Conduct/Oppositional Defiant
- Depression

- Eating
- Impulse Control Issues
- Substance Abuse
- Substance Dependence
- Trauma

ANGER AND EMOTIONAL DYSREGULATION

Dialectics:

- Having intense emotions and wanting to be calm. Skill: ***Square Breathing***
- Feeling out of control and wanting to be in control. Skill: ***Moment to Pause***
- Quick reactions and learning to be responsive. Skill: ***Feeling Not Acting***

Mindfulness:

Being in the moment can empower you to notice and intervene when you start to gear up emotionally.

Distress Tolerance:

These skills teach you to manage and tolerate strong emotions and crises without having to act on them.

Emotional Regulation:

By maintaining awareness of your emotional state, and pausing for a moment, you can focus on using a skill instead of acting out your emotions or impulses.

Interpersonal Effectiveness:

These skills can help the you avoid harming others emotionally or physically.

BRIEF VIGNETTE:

A 42-year-old female client is experiencing problems with anger. She yells at people who are driving near her. She gets so upset at work that she leaves abruptly and without permission. She throws things at family members but does not physically harm anyone. She is usually very upset with herself but reports having no control over her behavior.

Additional Client Information: _____

_____

_____

_____

SUGGESTED SKILLS:

- Mindfulness: ***Non-Judgmental***. Suspend evaluations about self and others.

- Distress Tolerance: ***Half-Smile***. Find something in your day or in your life that you can have a genuine half-smile about. When you have a half-smile you are a bit more relaxed.

- Emotional Regulation: ***TRUST***. **T**rust yourself, **R**edirect impulses and urges, **U**se your skills, act consistently with the way you want to be **S**een, **T**ame your emotions and reactions.

- Interpersonal Effectiveness: ***Four Horsemen***. Identify the four most destructive issues you bring into your relationships and use mindfulness and other skills to keep these forces out of your relationships.

OTHER SKILLS AND HOW YOU WOULD TEACH THEM:

_____

_____

_____

_____

_____

_____

_____

_____

_____

_____

_____

ANXIETY

Dialectics:

- Worrying a lot and wanting to be safe. Skill: ***Wise Mind***
- Hypersensitivity and being grounded in the body. Skill: ***Body Scan***
- Worst-case scenario and having options. Skill: ***Keeping It in Perspective***

Mindfulness:

Stay grounded in the current moment without getting caught up in the past or the future.

Distress Tolerance:

Reduce catastrophizing. Be willing to accept anxiety. Use skills to reduce frustration and pain.

Emotional Regulation:

Use skills to help reduce the intensity of emotions.

Interpersonal Effectiveness:

Continue to have healthy relationships even with anxiety.

BRIEF VIGNETTE:

A 27-year-old male is struggling with an inability to leave his house. He reports having panic attacks and worries that he is dying. He is fearful about being embarrassed or not being able to get out of a situation if there is a problem. This has been going on for about a year. Because of his anxiety, he has been getting in trouble at work and has a great deal of conflict in his marriage.

Additional Client Information: _____

_____

_____

_____

SUGGESTED SKILLS:

- *Mindfulness*: **One-Mindfully**. One thing at a time.
- *Distress Tolerance*: **Self-Soothe**. Self-soothe with all five of your senses: sight, sound, smell, taste, and touch.
- *Emotional Regulation*: **Opposite to Emotion**. Engage in the action that will bring into your awareness the opposite emotion to what you are feeling.
- *Interpersonal Effectiveness*: **DEAR WOMAN or MAN**. Use the acronym to **D**escribe what is wanted, **E**ncourage others, **A**sk, **R**einforce others, **W**illingness, **O**bserve, **M**indful, **A**ppear Confident, and **N**egotiate.

OTHER SKILLS AND HOW YOU WOULD TEACH THEM:

_____

_____

_____

_____

_____

_____

_____

_____

_____

_____

_____

BIPOLAR

Dialectics:

- Wanting to have the mania and avoid the depression. Skill: **Ride the Wave**
- Having fun and taking care of self. Skill: **MEDDSS**
- Energy and exhaustion. Skill: **EMOTIONS**

Mindfulness:

Staying in the present empowers you to move beyond previous mood swings and destructive behaviors associated with them.

Distress Tolerance:

These skills help you to manage your crises and negative moods.

Emotional Regulation:

You are able to track your emotions, engage in balanced self-care, and stay connected to your psychiatric prescriber.

Interpersonal Effectiveness:

Maintaining healthy relationships contributes to stability with this diagnosis.

BRIEF VIGNETTE:

A 37-year-old female reports a history of three previous manic episodes with accompanying hospitalizations. She also reports experiencing depression off and on throughout her life. A relapse of her depression seems to be indicated by her sleeping 10+ hours a night, calling in sick at work, and withdrawing from her family. She also reports using methamphetamine and alcohol to avoid the depression and keep the mania going.

Additional Client Information: _____

_____

_____

_____

SUGGESTED SKILLS:

- *Mindfulness*: **ONE MIND**. **O**ne thing at a time, here and **N**ow, be grounded in the **E**nvironment, be present in this one **M**oment, **I**ncrease senses to be firmly in the here and now, be **N**on-Judgmental of self and others, **D**escribe things in concrete, specific terms.

- *Distress Tolerance*: **Keep it in Perspective**. This is the marathon of crises and all of the other crises and difficulties have been training for this one. You are now in the best shape of your life. You are well experienced and can definitely deal effectively with this crisis.

- *Emotional Regulation*: **Love Dandelions**. Build an awareness and acceptance of parts of yourself that you don't like or that you find unattractive.

- *Interpersonal Effectiveness*: **Broken Record**. Be a broken record with yourself. Keep coming back to your needs.

OTHER SKILLS AND HOW YOU WOULD TEACH THEM:

_____

_____

_____

_____

_____

_____

_____

_____

_____

_____

CONDUCT/OPPOSITIONAL DEFIANT DISORDER (YOUTH)

Dialectics:

- Self-interest and relationships with others. Skill: ***Relationship Assumptions***
- Feeling good and acting in best interests. Skill: ***Feeling Not Acting***
- Short-term goals and long-term plans. Skill: ***Ride the Wave***

Mindfulness:

These skills can get you out of your head about what you think is going on and stay closer to your actual experiences.

Distress Tolerance:

These skills may be essential for self-regulation to help you stop destructive, harmful behavior.

Emotional Regulation:

You can benefit greatly from effectively getting to know and learning to manage your emotions.

Interpersonal Effectiveness:

With these difficulties you may struggle in relationships, particularly with authority figures. Interpersonal Effectiveness can increase confidence and competency.

BRIEF VIGNETTE:

A 13-year-old male harms animals and attends school only 75% of the time. He often ignores the directions of his teachers and parents. He gets upset with others and throws temper tantrums. He has gotten in trouble at school for getting revenge on other children whom he believes did things to harm him.

Additional Client Information: _____

_____

_____

_____

SUGGESTED SKILLS:

- <u>*Mindfulness*</u>: **Effectively**. Be as effective as you can in your life.
- <u>*Distress Tolerance*</u>: **Turning the Mind**. You are in the driver's seat with your mind, not just a passenger in your life. This includes thoughts, feelings, impulses, and even behavior.
- <u>*Emotional Regulation*</u>: **Lemonade**. Give yourself credit for your strengths and ability to survive difficulty.
- <u>*Interpersonal Effectiveness*</u>: **Turn the Tables/Pay It Forward**. Be reciprocal. Do things for other people. Do things for others even when you don't get anything back.

OTHER SKILLS AND HOW YOU WOULD TEACH THEM:

_____

_____

_____

_____

_____

_____

_____

_____

_____

_____

_____

_____

DEPRESSION

Dialectics:

- Hopelessness and optimism. Skill: ***Keeping it in Perspective***
- Pain and enjoyment. Skill: ***ACCEPTS***
- Past, present, and future. Skill: ***ONE MIND***

Mindfulness:

Being in the here and now reduces rumination about how it has always been this way and will always be this way.

Distress Tolerance:

These skills can help manage hopelessness and suicidal feelings.

Emotional Regulation:

The self-care embedded in these skills can be invaluable.

Interpersonal Effectiveness:

These skills can combat the low self-esteem associated with mood disorders so that you can be effective in your relationships.

BRIEF VIGNETTE:

A 21-year-old female reports that she sleeps 12–14 hours a day. She hasn't been eating much and has lost 20 pounds in the last two months. She has very few friends. She lost her job due to frequent absences and tardiness. She feels hopeless and wonders if life is worth living. She hasn't been suicidal in the past and there are no current concerns about lethal self-harm.

Additional Client Information: _____

_____

_____

_____

SUGGESTED SKILLS:

- *Mindfulness:* **Observe/Describe/Participate**. Just notice. Become aware of things in this one moment. Describe your experience in concrete, specific, non-judgmental terms. Engage fully and completely in each activity.

- *Distress Tolerance:* **Crisis Survival Network**. Have a list of people who support you and help you deal with difficulties. Have as many people as possible on the list and use them flexibly.

- *Emotional Regulation:* **EMOTIONS**. **E**xposure to emotions, be **M**indful of current emotions, **O**utline a plan to deal with emotions, **T**ake opposite action, **I**ncrease positive experiences, anticipate **O**bstacles and plan to overcome them, **N**otice what is going on, and **S**upport system.

- *Interpersonal Effectiveness:* **Relationship Mindfulness**. Identify generalizations, describe assumptions, suspend judgments, avoid jumping to conclusions, be self-empowering not self-defeating, use "One-Mindfulness," be non-judgmental, and participate effectively.

OTHER SKILLS AND HOW YOU WOULD TEACH THEM:

_____

_____

_____

_____

_____

_____

_____

_____

_____

_____

EATING

Dialectics:

- Indulgence and restraint. Skill: **IMPROVES**
- Control and ability to let go. Skill: **Repairs**
- Enjoyment and deprivation. Skill: **Wise Mind**

Mindfulness:

It is essential to stay present with the ritual of eating while being non-judgmental.

Distress Tolerance:

These are essential skills for managing the internal distress that may not be observable to others.

Emotional Regulation:

These skills can assist you in managing your emotions more effectively.

Interpersonal Effectiveness:

These skills can help the you and your support system to establish healthy communication.

BRIEF VIGNETTE:

A 13-year-old female engages in restrictive eating and binging and purging behavior. She is slightly underweight but not significantly. She does have an unrealistic body image. Her family is highly conflictual. She excels academically but doesn't have any close friends. She doesn't get involved in after-school or recreational activities.

Additional Client Information: _____

_____

_____

_____

SUGGESTED SKILLS:

- <u>Mindfulness</u>: **Square Breathing**. Breathe in while counting to four. Hold for four seconds. Exhale while counting to four. Repeat four times.
- <u>Distress Tolerance</u>: **Self-Soothe 1st Aid Kit**. Create a kit that is self-soothing and use when needed.
- <u>Emotional Regulation</u>: **BEHAVIOR**. **B**ehavior, **E**nvironment, **H**ealing vs. **H**urting, **A**ntecedents, **V**alues, **I**nterval, **O**utcome, and **R**einforcement.
- <u>Interpersonal Effectiveness</u>: **Relationship Thinking**. Reduce or eliminate black-and-white thinking. Foster dialectical thinking by seeing things from multiple viewpoints and holding a both/and perspective.

OTHER SKILLS AND HOW YOU WOULD TEACH THEM:

_____

_____

_____

_____

_____

_____

_____

_____

_____

IMPULSE CONTROL PROBLEMS

Dialectics:

- Right now and in a little while. Skill: ***TRUST***
- Willfulness and self-discipline. Skill: ***Willingness***
- Yes and no. Skill: ***DEAR WOMAN or MAN***

Mindfulness:

Staying in the moment helps you learn to be with your impulses without necessarily acting on them.

Distress Tolerance:

These skills give you something to do besides acting on an impulse. They can provide a replacement or a distraction.

Emotional Regulation:

Managing emotions effectively can reduce or eliminate impulsiveness. Using the moment-to-pause skill helps you have more control.

Interpersonal Effectiveness:

These skills can provide motivation to improve management of impulses.

BRIEF VIGNETTE:

A 16-year-old male can't seem to control himself. He drinks his parents' alcohol. He plays video games for hours. He gets upset at school, yelling and using obscenities. He has had one occasion of harming the family pet. He is suspected of graffiti in the neighborhood.

Additional Client Information: _____

_____

_____

_____

SUGGESTED SKILLS:

- *Mindfulness*: **Wise Mind**. Balancing Rational Mind and Emotional Mind to create Wise Mind.

- *Distress Tolerance*: **Willingness**. Willingness exercises are helpful in the middle of a crisis. Practice willingness to accept reality, a bad day, things not going your way, or to accept that you can't control others and the world around you.

- *Emotional Regulation*: **Ride the Wave**. Just like the tides that come and go and yet are always with us, so are our emotions and impulses. Some days are stormy and chaotic while other days are calmer. Imagine that you are riding the wave of your emotions. This can be envisioned as surfing, snowboarding, skiing, or skateboarding.

- *Interpersonal Effectiveness*: **GIVE**. Be **G**entle in relationships, show **I**nterest in others, **V**alidate others, and have an **E**asy Manner

OTHER SKILLS AND HOW YOU WOULD TEACH THEM:

_____

_____

_____

_____

_____

_____

_____

_____

_____

_____

_____

_____

SUBSTANCE ABUSE

Dialectics:

- Checking out and being present in life. Skill: ***Opposite to Emotions***
- Have fun and be responsible. Skill: ***Non-Judgmental***
- Trying to be in control and losing control. Skill: ***Wise Mind***

Mindfulness:

Staying in the moment can help you focus on the tasks at hand and reduce avoidance behaviors.

Distress Tolerance:

Effectively managing difficult situations can reduce the need for substances.

Emotional Regulation:

These skills can increase stability and life satisfaction.

Interpersonal Effectiveness:

By being more functional in your relationships you may find less need for substances.

BRIEF VIGNETTE:

A 24-year-old woman uses marijuana and alcohol a couple of times a week. She has missed work a couple of times in the last year. She has a job at which she seems to do well. Her home life is stable. She reports wanting more from life. She says she plans to go back to school but doesn't seem to get around to it. She sleeps a lot and eats more than she wants to. Her self-care seems impaired.

Additional Client Information: _____

_____

_____

_____

SUGGESTED SKILLS:

- _Mindfulness_: **Be Mindful**. Be mindful of using a skill, self-care, having healthy fun, and having a connection to your support system.
- _Distress Tolerance_: **IMPROVE**. Distract yourself with **I**magery of a beautiful or safe place, **M**eaning in your life, **P**rayer, **R**elaxation, **O**ne-Mindfully, **V**acation from the demands of your life, and **E**ncouragement to be effective
- _Emotional Regulation_: **Feeling Not Acting**. Use your "Moment to Pause" skill to identify and feel the impulse or urge. Choose a skill to manage it or tolerate it while doing nothing.
- _Interpersonal Effectiveness_: **Ignore**. Ignore self-judgments and judgments of others.

OTHER SKILLS AND HOW YOU WOULD TEACH THEM:

_____

_____

_____

_____

_____

_____

_____

_____

_____

SUBSTANCE DEPENDENCE

Dialectics:

- Denying reality and knowing the truth. Skill: ***BEHAVIOR***
- Deceiving self and others. Skill: ***Turtling***
- Persistent and giving up. Skill: ***Feeling Not Acting***

Mindfulness:

If you are struggling with addiction, you may spend very little time in the here and now. Mindfulness can be quite empowering and essential to establishing recovery.

Distress Tolerance:

These skills can be extremely useful to you because you may have very little tolerance for frustration or pain.

Emotional Regulation:

The intensity of your emotions can be overpowering and trigger relapses. You may a have a strong tendency to engage in impulsive behavior.

Interpersonal Effectiveness:

You may have impaired relationships due to your addiction and you can benefit greatly from these skills.

BRIEF VIGNETTE:

A 56-year-old male has been using alcohol, marijuana, and cocaine for most of his adult life. He has been through treatment before but could only maintain sobriety for a few months. He uses because it is "fun" and helps him feel "normal." He reports having cravings which he responds to by using.

Additional Client Information: _____

_____

_____

_____

SUGGESTED SKILLS:

- _Mindfulness_: **Moment to Pause**. Take a quick moment to check in with yourself on the inside, around you, and with any interactions in relationships.
- _Distress Tolerance_: **Radical Acceptance**. Focus on what you have control of: Your own thoughts, feelings, impulses, and behaviors. Let go of what you can't control: others and the world around you.
- _Emotional Regulation_: **MEDDSS**. **M**astery, **E**xercise, **D**iet, **D**rugs, **S**leep, and **S**pirituality
- _Interpersonal Effectiveness_: **Making Repairs**. Apologize sometimes, accept apologies from others, and be willing to let go and move on.

OTHER SKILLS AND HOW YOU WOULD TEACH THEM:

_____

_____

_____

_____

_____

_____

_____

_____

_____

_____

_____

TRAUMA

Dialectics:

- Disempowered and empowered. Skill: ***Half-Smile***
- Victim and survivor. Skill: ***Lemonade***
- Danger and safety. Skill: ***DEAR WOMAN or MAN***

Mindfulness:

This can help you stop reliving the traumatic event(s). It also helps to acknowledge that the event is not occurring in the present moment.

Distress Tolerance:

These skills can help to reduce hypervigilance as well as to manage crises you experience.

Emotional Regulation:

These skills can be used to manage the emotional intensity associated with this diagnosis.

Interpersonal Effectiveness:

These skills can help you to have appropriate assertiveness, self-respect, and investment in relationships.

BRIEF VIGNETTE:

A 15-year-old female was sexually molested by a next door neighbor when she was 11 years-old. She is having trouble sleeping and thinks a lot about the event. She is quite jumpy and cries a lot. She knows she is missing out on many of the typical teenage activities but she can't trust other people.

Additional Client Information: _____

_____

_____

_____

SUGGESTED SKILLS:

- *Mindfulness*: **Turtling**. Take care of yourself like a turtle. Retreat inside for safety sometimes, go slowly and methodically, protect yourself but don't be aggressive, be adaptive in a variety of situations, use your hard outer shell to let others' judgments roll off your back, and persistently get yourself back in balance.

- *Distress Tolerance*: ACCEPTS. Distract yourself with **A**ctivities, **C**ontributing, **C**omparisons, **E**motions, **P**ushing Away, **T**houghts, and **S**ensations.

- *Emotional Regulation*: **Build + Emotions**. Balance negative emotions and experiences by increasing positive emotions and experiences. Do pleasant things that are possible now.

- *Interpersonal Effectiveness*: **FAST**. Be **F**air to self, **A**pologize less, **S**tick to your values, and be **T**ruthful with yourself.

OTHER SKILLS AND HOW YOU WOULD TEACH THEM:

_____

_____

_____

_____

_____

_____

_____

_____

_____

_____

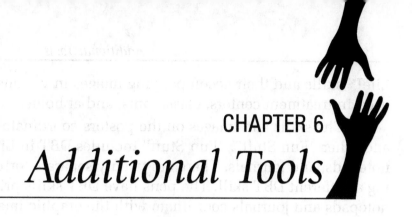

CHAPTER 6
Additional Tools

DBT IN LIFE PRODUCTS

Developing Balanced Travels in Life™ (D.B.T. in Life ™) products have been created by Cathy Moonshine, Ph.D., MAC, CADC III and are distributed through Moonshine-Consulting.com. These products are designed to educate youth and adults about how DBT skills can enhance their ability to effectively deal with stress and troubles. These skills can be very useful, not only for individuals with significant problems and difficulties, but also in optimizing functioning and life satisfaction for individuals who are relatively well-adjusted and self-actualized.

D.B.T. in Life ™ is about the ability to tolerate and effectively manage life's inherent confusions, paradoxes, and ironies. It is about avoiding extremes, such as "people are either with me or against me," "all or nothing," "lots of work and no play," "it's all about me and who cares what others want," or unhealthy lifestyles that lack important elements of self-care.

Being balanced in life is about a "both/and" perspective instead of an "either/or" perspective. Individuals can:

- Have friends and families who support them while sometimes disagreeing with them.
- Work hard and enjoy life.
- Take care of themselves and still help others.
- Engage in problematic behavior and maintain healthy self-care.

People generally experience more life satisfaction, sustain healthier relationships, and achieve more of their goals when they are able to balance the dialectics in their lives.

DBT in Life™ products include an annual garden calendar, games, posters, and other "Fun Stuff." The annual calendar is a full-color calendar with pictures of Moonshine Gardens in Portland, Oregon. Each month contains a different DBT skill, reminding folks to use their skills on a regular basis. The calendar will appeal more to mature audiences than the games, which include a deck of playing cards, Bingo Cards, a Bonanza Dice Game, and a board game. The games provide opportunities to have fun and appeal to all three learning styles while reinforcing learning the DBT skills. The posters are graphic images of each of the DBT in

Life™ skills and their accompanying images in various sizes. These posters can be used in treatment centers, classrooms, and at home.

The skills and images on the posters coordinate with graphics in the games and other "Fun Stuff". "Fun Stuff" includes DBT in Life™ fortune cookies, pens, notepads, and journals. There are twenty separate fortunes with each one including a different DBT skill. The pens have DBT skills printed on them and the notepads and journals coordinate with the graphic images in the games and posters. All of the "Fun Stuff" from the DBT in Life™ store can be given at the end of a session, as an incentive for completing diary cards, or as a reward for the client demonstrating or explaining how he used a skill.

DBT in Life™ products are designed to teach, reinforce learning, and make using DBT skills fun. They can be used in a variety of settings including:

- Individual sessions
- Group sessions
- Recreation activities
- Unstructured time in the therapeutic community
- In the classroom
- At home with family and friends

Products are designed to appeal to all three learning styles: kinesthetic, auditory, and visual. Another important component for learning is having fun and DBT in Life™ products are colorful, multi-faceted, and fast-paced. Having a sense of humor enhances many experiences in life, including learning. All of the different tactile and visual components of the products capture clients' attention. When learning is easy, fun, relevant, and stimulating clients are more likely to remember what they have learned and apply it in their day-to-day life.

DIARY CARDS

This is the way that clinicians ask clients to track how often they are using DBT skills. Any way that the client can reliably track the frequency of skill use can work. This can include recording the use of skills in a checkbook register, journal, day planner, mp3 player, e-mail or calendar program, or other electronic methods. When a client tracks how often a skill is used, he will use the skill more often.

At first most clients will have difficulty in consistently remembering to track their skill use. It is important to gently hold them accountable and to explore ways to improve their tracking efforts. If clients don't complete their cards between sessions taking a few minutes to fill out the card during the session is a useful way to reinforce the importance of tracking skill use. If filling out the cards doesn't make sense in session, have the client talk in detail about how he used the skill three to five times since the previous session.

The diary cards also help to keep the clinician organized. When a client brings diary cards to the session, the clinician knows which skills they have taught. This helps the clinician to stay on track and to have a sense of what skill to teach next. Reviewing the diary cards with the client also provides an opportunity to hear how the client is using the skills and to provide positive reinforcement, coaching, or corrective feedback. It also provides a time for working through resistance, fears, concerns, or barriers.

Typically there are skills that don't resonate with a particular client. For the most part this is reasonable; however some clients may be avoiding learning or using a specific skill that would be in their best interest. In this case the clinician assists the client to see the usefulness of the skill and to effectively deal with obstacles.

In the next few pages are some examples of different types of diary cards. The first example is for use with lined note cards or index cards. Using colored index cards allows for color-coding each module. The client writes out the definition of the skill on the lined part of the card. The reverse, unlined side of the card would be sectioned off into seven parts to record skills used each day. Writing out what the skill means to him gives the client an opportunity to put the skill into his own language. If the client gets it wrong or misinterprets the skill it provides the clinician with a "teachable moment" to clarify and give corrective feedback.

An additional benefit of having clients write out the skill is that it will stick better in their minds. They will remember the skills more easily because they have written them down. It is recommended that cards be kept in places where the clients will see them every day such as near the coffee pot, under the computer keyboard, or on the nightstand. Clients can take a few minutes every day to fill out their cards. In the beginning filling out the cards daily will be a challenge for most clients. Work with clients to achieve a regular pattern of filling out the cards.

Many clients will begin using skills but be inconsistent in their documentation on the cards. These clients may tell their clinicians that they are using the skills without filling out the cards and ask to be exempt from this requirement. It may be tempting for some clinicians to let their clients "off the hook" because they want to reward the client's hard work. These same clinicians may have their own resistance to homework and don't want the responsibility of checking the cards so they grant the client's request. This is a misstep. Clients can remember to practice a couple of skills for a week or two but most clients can't remember multiple skills for several weeks. Clinicians are strongly encouraged to find ways to have clients track their skills for the client's benefit as well as to help in the organization of the clinical process.

DIARY CARDS ON NOTE CARDS

- Mindfulness: Blue Cards
- Distress Tolerance: Yellow Cards
- Emotional Regulation: Green Cards
- Interpersonal Effectiveness: Pink Cards

Front of Note Card:

Mindfulness Skill:
Definition
_____
_____
_____

Back of Note Card:

Sunday	Monday	Tuesday	Wednesday	Thursday	Friday	Saturday

Front of Note Card:

Distress Tolerance Skill:
Definition
_____
_____
_____

Back of Note Card:

Sunday	Monday	Tuesday	Wednesday	Thursday	Friday	Saturday

Front of Note Card:

Emotional Regulation Skill:

Definition

_____

_____

_____

Back of Note Card:

Sunday	Monday	Tuesday	Wednesday	Thursday	Friday	Saturday

Front of Note Card:

Interpersonal Effectiveness Skill:

Definition

_____

_____

_____

Back of Note Card:

Sunday	Monday	Tuesday	Wednesday	Thursday	Friday	Saturday

The second example of diary cards is next. This is a comprehensive card that takes a full page. An alternative would be to print the card in landscape format. Either of these cards can be made in Microsoft Excel, Word, or another word processing program by using the "Create Table" option. This example allows four slots for skills in each of the four categories. These can be left blank if a variety of skills are taught to different clients or the cards can be pre-printed if a program teaches the same skills.

The example has a space on the back of the cards for clients to explore their impulses, feelings, and behaviors along with noting when they used the skills. Hopefully clients will build the insight that they can use their skills to effectively cope with their impulses, feelings, and behaviors. They may also see that when they have days with out-of-control impulses, feelings, and behaviors they probably aren't using their skills.

For an illustration of how this might work see the completed card on the following pages. Pay particular attention to Monday and Friday. On Monday the client had strong impulses, feelings, and behaviors but either didn't use the skills or thought they wouldn't work. On Friday the client experienced mild impulses, feelings, and behaviors. On this day the client used the skills. Talking about this card in therapy would help both the client and the clinician to see that the skills were helpful in minimizing the problematic impulses, feelings, and behaviors.

These are not the only options for diary cards. Clinicians are encouraged to think about their audience, make their diary cards user friendly, be creative, and take advantage of available technology whenever possible.

Too often diary cards are not implemented or maintained in the DBT process. The benefits of DBT will be diminished by foregoing a regular diary card regimen. If you can identify client and clinician barriers to using the cards and lower them, it will maximize the benefit of the skills and the entire DBT therapeutic process.

Full Page
DBT DIARY CARD

DBT Skills	Mon	Tues	Wed	Thur	Fri	Sat	Sun	Total
MINDFULNESS								
DISTRESS TOLERANCE								
EMOTIONAL REGULATION								
INTERPERSONAL EFFECTIVENESS								

Comments:

		Mon	Tues	Wed	Thur	Fri	Sat	Sun
IMPULSES TO*								
FEELINGS*								
BEHAVIORS*								
DBT SKILLS*								

Rating Scale: 0–5*	**Rate DBT Skills
• Impulses To • Feelings • Behaviors *5 is the highest	0 = Not thought about or used 1 = Thought about, didn't want to use skill 2 = Thought about, didn't use, but wanted to 3 = Tried to use skill, couldn't use it 4 = Tried to use skill, didn't help 5 = Used skill, it helped

Full Page
DBT DIARY CARD

DBT Skills	*Mon*	*Tues*	*Wed*	*Thur*	*Fri*	*Sat*	*Sun*	*Total*
MINDFULNESS								
Wise Mind	3	5	0	1		6		**15**
Turtling	0	0	2	2		4		**8**
Non-Judgmental	20+	20+	20+	20+		20+		**100+**
ONE MIND	0	0	0	0		0		**0**
DISTRESS TOLERANCE								
Crisis Survival Network	1	5	8	3		12		**29**
Self-Soothe First Aid Kit	6	9	23	13		1		**52**
Half-Smile	5	9	3	0		1		**18**
IMPROVES	0	0	0	0		1		**1**
EMOTIONAL REGULATION								
MEDDS	1	1	1	1		1		**5**
Love Dandelions	0	0	1	2		0		**3**
Opposite to Emotions	1	0	0	0		0		**1**
TRUST	2	0	0	6		1		**9**
INTERPERSONAL EFFECTIVENESS								
Making Repairs	0	0	0	0		0		**0**
GIVE	1	0	1	0		0		**2**
FAST	0	0	0	0		0		**0**
DEAR MAN	2	3	5	9		8		**27**

Comments:

	Mon	*Tues*	*Wed*	*Thur*	*Fri*	*Sat*	*Sun*
IMPULSES TO*							
Drop Out	4	2	1	2	1	1	5
Use AOD	5	1	1	3	2	2	4
Sex	5	3	1	5	0	3	3
Self-Harm	5	4	1	2	0	4	2
Sucide	3	4	1	1	0	5	2
FEELINGS*							
Anger	4	2	2	1	1	1	1
Sadness	5	3	1	3	0	2	1
Hopelessness	5	4	1	2	0	3	2
Shame	3	4	2	4	3	4	4
Loneliness	5	1	2	3	1	5	3
BEHAVIORS*							
No Show	2	2	1	2	0	1	0
Drink	5	1	2	1	0	0	0
Get High	5	0	2	2	0	2	0
Sex	5	2	1	3	1	0	0
Burn Self	0	3	1	1	0	1	0
DBT SKILLS*							
Non-Judgmental	0	5	3	3	5	4	5
Self-Soothe First Aid Kit	0	3	4	3	4	5	5
Crisis Survival	1	4	3	3	5	3	5
DEAR MAN	1	4	5	3	5	5	5

Rating Scale: 0–5*	**Rate DBT Skills
• Impulses To • Feelings • Behaviors *5 is the highest	0 = Not thought about or used 1 = Thought about, didn't want to use skill 2 = Thought about, didn't use, but wanted to 3 = Tried to use skill, couldn't use it 4 = Tried to use skill, didn't help 5 = Used skill, it helped

CHAIN ANALYSIS

DBT is a very complex model and one of the most intricate parts is chain analysis. Creating a chain analysis is similar to conducting a CBT functional analysis. In its simplest form chain analysis is about figuring out what led up to the client engaging in problem behaviors. Suicide attempts, self-harm incidents, harming others, using alcohol and other drugs, gambling, risky sexual behavior, engaging in out-of-control or restrictive eating, excessive exercise, raging, dangerous driving, criminal behavior, delinquency, bullying, graffiti, or property destruction are only a few examples of problem behaviors.

The metaphor of the chain analysis is that of the links of a chain or the chain of events that led to the problem behavior. For more complex examples visit http://www.behavioraltech.com or find the copyrighted form by checking the DBT literature or Dr. Linehan's publications.

In this text a more streamlined process is presented. Chain analyses are completed by the client, either with the clinician or as homework, and they begin by identifying the problem behavior. Some clients then figure things out by going backwards looking for what set off the chain of events. Other clients already have a sense of what started the process so they go to the beginning and work forward.

Chain analyses in their simplest form entail internal vulnerability, external triggers, and problem behavior. Based on these three components a solution analysis is completed. The solution analysis asks the clients to identify one to three skills they could use to more effectively deal with difficulties.

See the blank form on the next page for a graphic example of how a chain analysis can be formatted. This simple form is a good first step in learning to understand the chain of events leading to a problem behavior.

SIMPLE CHAIN ANALYSIS

What problem behavior are you analyzing?

_____

Now you are going to look at the chain of events that resulted in the problem behavior. These are referred to as links in the chain of events.

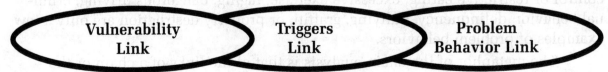

1. Vulnerability Link: In what ways was I vulnerable?

   • May be internal, such as thoughts, judgments, feelings, or impulses.

   • May be environmental, such as events, people, places, or situations.

   • May be interpersonal, such as difficult interactions with family or friends.

   ┌───┐
   │   │
   │   │
   │   │
   │   │
   └───┘

2. Triggers Link: What were the internal, environmental, and interpersonal triggers?

   • May be my actions, thoughts, judgments, feelings, or impulses, or people, places, situations, events, or interactions.

   ┌───┐
   │   │
   │   │
   │   │
   │   │
   └───┘

3. Problem Behavior Link: What was the problem behavior and any related behavior?

   • These are behavioral expressions that are problematic, harmful, or destructive.

   ┌───┐
   │   │
   │   │
   │   │
   │   │
   └───┘

SOLUTION ANALYSIS WORKSHEET

Now it is time to explore each link to come up with more effective response strategies.

Vulnerability Link: _____

Solution #1: _____

Solution #2: _____

Solution #3: _____

Triggers Link: _____

Solution #1: _____

Solution #2: _____

Solution #3: _____

Problem Behavior Link: _____

Solution #1: _____

Solution #2: _____

Solution #3: _____

SIMPLE CHAIN ANALYSIS

What problem behavior are you analyzing?

Beating up my younger brother.

Now you are going to look at the chain of events that resulted in the problem behavior. These are referred to as links in the chain of events.

Vulnerability Link	Triggers Link	Problem Behavior Link

1. Vulnerability Link: In what ways was I vulnerable?

Being bored. Doing nothing. Staring at the TV for hours changing channels. Staying up all night playing video games. Being late for school and falling asleep in class. Not doing my homework. Getting in trouble.

2. Triggers Link: What were the internal, environmental, and interpersonal triggers?

Thinking about other kids having fun, like those on my team in my video game. Remembering how I made it to my current level by being strong and beating up other characters and hurting them seriously. Some friends telling me they were going to ditch class to smoke some pot and go home to drink their parents' booze. Choosing to ditch class and go with them.

3. Problem Behavior Link: What was the problem behavior and any related behavior?

Getting high, drinking, and then deciding to beat up my younger brother.

SOLUTION ANALYSIS WORKSHEET

Now it is time to explore each link to come up with more effective response strategies.

Vulnerability Link: Being bored.

Solution #1: **Build positive emotional experiences**

Solution #2: **ACCEPTS**

Triggers Link: Thinking about other kids having fun, especially those I play video games with.

Solution #1: **Turning the Mind**

Solution #2: **Ride the Wave**

Problem Behavior Link: Beating up my younger brother.

Solution #1: **Ride the Wave**

Solution #2: **ACCEPTS**

SIMPLE CHAIN ANALYSIS

What problem behavior are you analyzing?

Sleeping all the time and not eating.

Now you are going to look at the chain of events that resulted in the problem behavior. These are referred to as links in the chain of events.

Vulnerability Link   **Triggers Link**   **Problem Behavior Link**

1. Vulnerability Link: In what ways was I vulnerable?

No energy, feeling hopeless and not wanting to have to take meds the rest of my life. Forgetting to take my meds and nothing bad happened. Ruminating about how exhausted I am.

2. Triggers Link: What were the internal, environmental, and interpersonal triggers?

Spending time on the Internet reading about how Tom Cruise and others say that we shouldn't take medication. Also, canceling plans, not answering my phone, running out of food and not going to the grocery store for more. Deciding not to take my meds, unplugging my phone, and still not buying food.

3. Problem Behavior Link: What was the problem behavior and any related behavior?

Sleeping nearly 20 hours a day, losing weight and being non-responsive to my family's attempts to support me.

SOLUTION ANALYSIS WORKSHEET

Now it is time to explore each link to come up with more effective response strategies.

Vulnerability Link: No energy, feeling hopeless.

Solution #1: **MEDDSS**

Solution #2: **Body Scan**

Solution #3: **Half-Smile**

Triggers Link: Running out of food and not going to grocery store.

Solution #1: **Turtling**

Solution #2: **MEDDSS**

Problem Behavior Link: Sleeping nearly 20 hours a day.

Solution #1: **Turtling**

Solution #2: **Wise Mind**

Solution #3: **Crisis Survival Network**

If clients have the intellectual ability and motivation to invest in a more in-depth process there is a second chain analysis form that adds two additional steps. Staying with the metaphor of a chain of events or the links in a chain, a connecting link has been added between vulnerability and trigger, and another between trigger and problem behavior. Connecting links are half-steps between vulnerability and trigger, as well as between trigger and problem behavior. The most important part of the connecting links is that they provide two additional opportunities for solutions (see the blank in-depth chain analysis form).

Beyond the blank form are examples of in-depth chain analyses, one for each of the Axis I diagnoses explored in Chapter 5.

IN-DEPTH CHAIN ANALYSIS

What problem behavior are you analyzing?

Now we are going to look at the chain of events that resulted in the problem behavior. These are referred to as links in the chain of events.

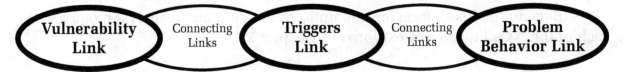

1. Vulnerability Link: In what ways was I vulnerable?

   • May be internal, such as thoughts, judgments, feelings, or impulses.

   • May be environmental, such as events, person, places, or situations.

   • May be interpersonal, such as difficult interactions with family or friends.

2. Connecting Links: What connected my vulnerability and triggers?

   • May be my actions, thoughts, judgments, feelings, or impulses, or people, places, situations, events, or interactions.

3. Triggers Link: What were the internal, environmental, and interpersonal triggers?

   • May be my actions, thoughts, judgments, feelings, or impulses, or people, places, situations, events, or interactions.

4. Connecting Links: What connected my triggers with the problem behavior?

   • May be my actions, thoughts, judgments, feelings, or impulses, or people, places, situations, events, or interactions.

5. Problem Behavior Link: What was the problem behavior and any related behavior?

   • These are behavioral expressions that are problematic, harmful, or destructive.

SOLUTION ANALYSIS WORKSHEET

Now it is time to explore each link to come up with more effective response strategies.

Vulnerability Link: _____

Solution #1: _____

Solution #2: _____

Solution #3: _____

Connecting Link: _____

Solution #1: _____

Solution #2: _____

Solution #3: _____

Triggers Link: _____

Solution #1: _____

Solution #2: _____

Solution #3: _____

Connecting Link: _____

Solution #1: _____

Solution #2: _____

Solution #3: _____

Problem Behavior Link: _____

Solution #1: _____

Solution #2: _____

Solution #3: _____

IN-DEPTH CHAIN ANALYSIS

What problem behavior are you analyzing?

Losing control of my anger, throwing things, and putting my fist through the wall.

Now you are going to look at the chain of events that resulted in the problem behavior. These are referred to as links in the chain of events.

1. Vulnerability Link: In what ways was I vulnerable?

Really stressed out about work and things at home.

2. Connecting Links: What connected my vulnerability and triggers?

Seems like I am up all night thinking about all I have to do.

3. Triggers Link: What were the internal, environmental, and interpersonal triggers?

Having another project assigned me at work. Then my boss told me that she was disappointed with my performance on the last project.

4. Connecting Links: What connected my triggers with the problem behavior?

Everybody seems to need something from me. I never seem to get a break.

5. Problem Behavior Link: What was the problem behavior and any related behavior?

Putting my fist through the wall.

SOLUTION ANALYSIS WORKSHEET

Now it is time to explore each link to come up with more effective response strategies.

Vulnerability Link: <u>Really stressed out.</u>

Solution #1: **<u>Ride the Wave</u>**

Solution #2: **<u>ACCEPTS</u>**

Solution #3: **<u>Body Scan</u>**

Connecting Link: <u>Up all night.</u>

Solution #1: **<u>Ride the Wave</u>**

Solution #2: **<u>ABC</u>**

Triggers Link: <u>My boss was disappointed with my performance.</u>

Solution #1: **<u>ABC</u>**

Solution #2: **<u>Body Scan</u>**

Solution #3: **<u>ACCEPTS</u>**

Connecting Link: <u>I never seem to get a break.</u>

Solution #1: **<u>ABC</u>**

Solution #2: **<u>Ride the Wave</u>**

Solution #3: **<u>Body Scan</u>**

Problem Behavior Link: <u>Putting my fist through the wall.</u>

Solution #1: **<u>TRUST</u>**

Solution #2: **<u>Ride the Wave</u>**

Solution #3: **<u>ABC</u>**

IN-DEPTH CHAIN ANALYSIS

What problem behavior are you analyzing?

Couldn't leave the house for three days straight.

Now you are going to look at the chain of events that resulted in the problem behavior. These are referred to as links in the chain of events.

1. Vulnerability Link: In what ways was I vulnerable?

I startle easily. I am very concerned about being embarrassed.

2. Connecting Links: What connected my vulnerability and triggers?

My heart started racing when I thought of leaving my house.

3. Triggers Link: What were the internal, environmental, and interpersonal triggers?

My friend called and said she wouldn't be meeting me at the event.

4. Connecting Links: What connected my triggers with the problem behavior?

I realized that I would be completely alone in a big group.

5. Problem Behavior Link: What was the problem behavior and any related behavior?

Stayed at home for three days straight. Didn't answer the phone or respond to e-mails.

SOLUTION ANALYSIS WORKSHEET

Now it is time to explore each link to come up with more effective response strategies.

Vulnerability Link: <u>I startle easily.</u>

Solution #1: **<u>Square Breathing</u>**

Solution #2: **<u>Self-Soothe First Aid Kit</u>**

Connecting Link: <u>My heart started racing when I thought of leaving my house.</u>

Solution #1: **<u>Self-Soothe First Aid Kit</u>**

Solution #2: **<u>ONE MIND</u>**

Triggers Link: <u>My friend called and said she wouldn't be meeting me at the event.</u>

Solution #1: **<u>Square Breathing</u>**

Solution #2: **<u>Dealing with Difficult People</u>**

Connecting Link: <u>I realized that I would be completely alone in a big group.</u>

Solution #1: **<u>Dealing with Difficult People</u>**

Solution #2: **<u>Square Breathing</u>**

Solution #3: **<u>Self-Soothe First Aid Kit</u>**

Problem Behavior Link: <u>Stayed at home for three days straight. Didn't answer the phone or respond to e-mails.</u>

Solution #1: **<u>Self-Soothe First Aid Kit</u>**

Solution #2: **<u>Square Breathing</u>**

Solution #3: **<u>Dealing with Difficult People</u>**

IN-DEPTH CHAIN ANALYSIS

What problem behavior are you analyzing?

 Bought a car on my credit card and painted it Pepto-Bismol pink while I was manic.

Now you are going to look at the chain of events that resulted in the problem behavior. These are referred to as links in the chain of events.

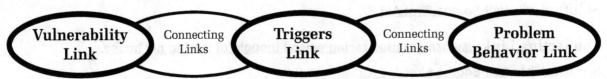

1. Vulnerability Link: In what ways was I vulnerable?

> **Not sleeping.**

2. Connecting Links: What connected my vulnerability and triggers?

> **Enjoy the energy and creativity.**

3. Triggers Link: What were the internal, environmental, and interpersonal triggers?

> **Stopped taking my medications.**

4. Connecting Links: What connected my triggers with the problem behavior?

> **Didn't tell my family or my doctor that I stopped taking my meds.**

5. Problem Behavior Link: What was the problem behavior and any related behavior?

> **Bought a car on my credit card and painted it Pepto-Bismol pink while I was manic.**

SOLUTION ANALYSIS WORKSHEET

Now it is time to explore each link to come up with more effective response strategies.

Vulnerability Link: <u>Not sleeping.</u>

Solution #1: <u>**MEDDSS**</u>

Solution #2: <u>**Willingness**</u>

Connecting Link: <u>Enjoy the energy and creativity.</u>

Solution #1: <u>**Getting to Know My Emotions**</u>

Solution #2: <u>**MEDDSS**</u>

Triggers Link: <u>Stopped taking my medications.</u>

Solution #1: <u>**MEDDSS**</u>

Connecting Link: <u>Didn't tell my family or my doctor that I stopped taking my meds.</u>

Solution #1: <u>**MEDDSS**</u>

Solution #2: <u>**Crisis Survival Network**</u>

Solution #3: <u>**Willingness**</u>

Problem Behavior Link: <u>Bought a car on my credit card and painted it Pepto-Bismol pink while I was manic.</u>

Solution #1: <u>**MEDDSS**</u>

Solution #2: <u>**Crisis Survival Network**</u>

Solution #3: <u>**Repairs**</u>

IN-DEPTH CHAIN ANALYSIS

What problem behavior are you analyzing?

 Getting in trouble for hurting animals.

Now you are going to look at the chain of events that resulted in the problem behavior. These are referred to as links in the chain of events.

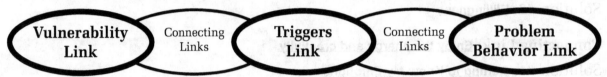

1. Vulnerability Link: In what ways was I vulnerable?

> **Really, really mad.**

2. Connecting Links: What connected my vulnerability and triggers?

> **Overheard another kid talking about me.**

3. Triggers Link: What were the internal, environmental, and interpersonal triggers?

> **Got in a fight during recess.**

4. Connecting Links: What connected my triggers with the problem behavior?

> **Got in-school suspension for three days. Parents threatened me with military school.**

5. Problem Behavior Link: What was the problem behavior and any related behavior?

> **Getting in trouble for hurting animals.**

SOLUTION ANALYSIS WORKSHEET

Now it is time to explore each link to come up with more effective response strategies.

Vulnerability Link: <u>Really, really mad.</u>

Solution #1: <u>Wise Mind</u>

Solution #2: <u>Opposite to Emotion</u>

Solution #3: <u>Turning the Mind</u>

Connecting Link: <u>Overheard another kid talking about me.</u>

Solution #1: <u>Opposite to Emotions</u>

Solution #2: <u>Turning the Mind</u>

Triggers Link: <u>Got in a fight during recess.</u>

Solution #1: <u>BEHAVIOR</u>

Solution #2: <u>Turning the Mind</u>

Connecting Link: <u>Got in-school suspension for three days. Parents threatened me with military school.</u>

Solution #1: <u>Keeping It In Perspective</u>

Solution #2: <u>Turning the Mind</u>

Solution #3: <u>Opposite to Emotions</u>

Problem Behavior Link: <u>Getting in trouble for hurting animals.</u>

Solution #1: <u>Keeping It In Perspective</u>

Solution #2: <u>Turning the Mind</u>

Solution #3: <u>Opposite to Emotions</u>

IN-DEPTH CHAIN ANALYSIS

What problem behavior are you analyzing?

 Not getting out of bed for several days.

Now you are going to look at the chain of events that resulted in the problem behavior. These are referred to as links in the chain of events.

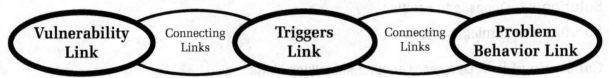

1. Vulnerability Link: In what ways was I vulnerable?

> **Believing my life is hopeless.**

2. Connecting Links: What connected my vulnerability and triggers?

> **No energy and nothing to do.**

3. Triggers Link: What were the internal, environmental, and interpersonal triggers?

> **Stopped taking medications and going to therapy appointments.**

4. Connecting Links: What connected my triggers with the problem behavior?

> **Didn't have any food in the house. Didn't think anyone would notice that I wasn't around.**

5. Problem Behavior Link: What was the problem behavior and any related behavior?

> **Didn't get out of bed for four days straight except to go to the bathroom.**

SOLUTION ANALYSIS WORKSHEET

Now it is time to explore each link to come up with more effective response strategies.

Vulnerability Link: <u>Believing my life is hopeless.</u>

Solution #1: <u>Turtling</u>

Solution #2: <u>Non-Judgmental</u>

Solution #3: <u>ABC</u>

Connecting Link: <u>No energy and nothing to do.</u>

Solution #1: <u>ABC</u>

Solution #2: <u>Turtling</u>

Solution #3: <u>Self-Soothe 1st Aid Kit</u>

Triggers Link: <u>Stopped taking medications and going to therapy appointments.</u>

Solution #1: <u>Turtling</u>

Solution #2: <u>ABC</u>

Solution #3: <u>Four Horsemen</u>

Connecting Link: <u>Didn't have any food in the house. Didn't think anyone would notice that I wasn't around.</u>

Solution #1: <u>Four Horsemen</u>

Solution #2: <u>Self-Soothe First Aid Kit</u>

Problem Behavior Link: <u>Didn't get out of bed for four days straight except to go to the bathroom.</u>

Solution #1: <u>Turtling</u>

Solution #2: <u>ABC</u>

Solution #3: <u>Four Horsemen</u>

IN-DEPTH CHAIN ANALYSIS

What problem behavior are you analyzing?

My eating is out of control.

Now you are going to look at the chain of events that resulted in the problem behavior. These are referred to as links in the chain of events.

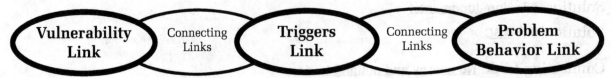

1. Vulnerability Link: In what ways was I vulnerable?

> I feel very sad and lonely.

2. Connecting Links: What connected my vulnerability and triggers?

> Nothing to do. Bored. Can't seem to have any fun in life.

3. Triggers Link: What were the internal, environmental, and interpersonal triggers?

> Completely alone. No real friends who care about me.

4. Connecting Links: What connected my triggers with the problem behavior?

> Tried to go to a dance at the community center but it was closed. Didn't find out until I got all the way over there. Felt like people were laughing at me when I arrived and found it wasn't happening.

5. Problem Behavior Link: What was the problem behavior and any related behavior?

> Went home and ate two gallons of ice cream, a couple of bags of potato chips, and countless candy bars.

SOLUTION ANALYSIS WORKSHEET

Now it is time to explore each link to come up with more effective response strategies.

Vulnerability Link: <u>**Vulnerability Link: I feel very sad and lonely.**</u>

Solution #1: <u>**Wise Mind**</u>

Solution #2: <u>**Lemonade**</u>

Solution #3: <u>**Turning the Mind**</u>

Connecting Link: <u>**Nothing to do. Bored. Can't seem to have any fun in life.**</u>

Solution #1: <u>**Building Positive Experiences**</u>

Solution #2: <u>**Effectively**</u>

Solution #3: <u>**Participate**</u>

Triggers Link: <u>**Completely alone. No real friends who care about me.**</u>

Solution #1: <u>**Effectively**</u>

Solution #2: <u>**IMPROVE**</u>

Solution #3: <u>**Turning the Mind**</u>

Connecting Link: <u>**Tried to go to a dance at the community center but it was closed.**</u>

Solution #1: <u>**Turning the Mind**</u>

Solution #2: <u>**IMPROVE**</u>

Solution #3: <u>**Effectively**</u>

Problem Behavior Link: <u>**Went home and ate two gallons of ice cream, a couple of bags of potato chips, and countless candy bars.**</u>

Solution #1: <u>**Effectively**</u>

Solution #2: <u>**Mindful Eating**</u>

Solution #3: <u>**Lemonade**</u>

IN-DEPTH CHAIN ANALYSIS

What problem behavior are you analyzing?

 Doing whatever I want which included having an anonymous sexual encounter.

Now you are going to look at the chain of events that resulted in the problem behavior. These are referred to as links in the chain of events.

| Vulnerability Link | Connecting Links | Triggers Link | Connecting Links | Problem Behavior Link |

1. Vulnerability Link: In what ways was I vulnerable?

> Bored, I was so bored. I thought about some things I could do but I rejected all of them. They seemed so boring.

2. Connecting Links: What connected my vulnerability and triggers?

> Nothing to do. Didn't reach out to my support system.

3. Triggers Link: What were the internal, environmental, and interpersonal triggers?

> Drove by a club that I used to go to when I was having a lot of sexual encounters.

4. Connecting Links: What connected my triggers with the problem behavior?

> Parked my car, went in, saw some old friends. Started drinking.

5. Problem Behavior Link: What was the problem behavior and any related behavior?

> Left the club with two people I didn't know. Had sex with them without using a condom.

SOLUTION ANALYSIS WORKSHEET

Now it is time to explore each link to come up with more effective response strategies.

Vulnerability Link: <u>Vulnerability Link: Bored, I was so bored.</u>

Solution #1: <u>Wise Mind</u>

Solution #2: <u>Love Dandelions</u>

Solution #3: <u>EMOTIONS</u>

Connecting Link: <u>Nothing to do.</u>

Solution #1: <u>Love Dandelions</u>

Solution #2: <u>EMOTIONS</u>

Triggers Link: <u>Drove by a club that I used to go to.</u>

Solution #1: <u>Relationship Thinking</u>

Solution #2: <u>Love Dandelions</u>

Solution #3: <u>EMOTIONS</u>

Connecting Link: <u>Saw some old friends.</u>

Solution #1: <u>Relationship Thinking</u>

Solution #2: <u>Wise Mind</u>

Solution #3: <u>Love Dandelions</u>

Problem Behavior Link: <u>Had sex without using a condom.</u>

Solution #1: <u>Relationship Thinking</u>

Solution #2: <u>Wise Mind</u>

Solution #3: <u>EMOTIONS</u>

IN-DEPTH CHAIN ANALYSIS

What problem behavior are you analyzing?

 __Getting high on the weekends.__

Now you are going to look at the chain of events that resulted in the problem behavior. These are referred to as links in the chain of events.

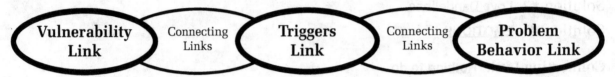

1. Vulnerability Link: In what ways was I vulnerable?

Was in a really good mood.

2. Connecting Links: What connected my vulnerability and triggers?

Thought that I had been doing really well with my self-care and decided I deserved a reward.

3. Triggers Link: What were the internal, environmental, and interpersonal triggers?

Called a friend to come over and bring a bottle of wine.

4. Connecting Links: What connected my triggers with the problem behavior?

Remembered that I had some pot stashed under the bed.

5. Problem Behavior Link: What was the problem behavior and any related behavior?

Started smoking pot and continued all weekend. Didn't do any of my self-care. Feel like I lost a whole weekend.

SOLUTION ANALYSIS WORKSHEET

Now it is time to explore each link to come up with more effective response strategies.

Vulnerability Link: <u>Vulnerability Link: Was in a really good mood.</u>
Solution #1: <u>ONE MIND</u>

Connecting Link: <u>Decided I deserved a reward.</u>
Solution #1: <u>Lemonade</u>
Solution #2: <u>ONE MIND</u>

Triggers Link: <u>Called a friend to come over and bring a bottle of wine.</u>
Solution #1: <u>Lemonade</u>
Solution #2: <u>ONE MIND</u>
Solution #3: <u>Pros and Cons</u>

Connecting Link: <u>Remembered that I had some pot stashed under the bed.</u>
Solution #1: <u>ONE MIND</u>
Solution #2: <u>Keeping It In Perspective</u>
Solution #3: <u>Pros and Cons</u>

Problem Behavior Link: <u>Started smoking pot.</u>
Solution #1: <u>Lemonade</u>
Solution #2: <u>ONE MIND</u>
Solution #3: <u>Keeping It In Perspective</u>

IN-DEPTH CHAIN ANALYSIS

What problem behavior are you analyzing?

 Can't stop drinking.

Now you are going to look at the chain of events that resulted in the problem behavior. These are referred to as links in the chain of events.

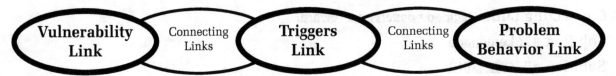

1. Vulnerability Link: In what ways was I vulnerable?

I feel so stressed out. Everything seems to be going wrong. Wondering why my life is so hard.

2. Connecting Links: What connected my vulnerability and triggers?

Was up all night thinking about how much my life sucks.

3. Triggers Link: What were the internal, environmental, and interpersonal triggers?

Car wouldn't start. Had to get a ride to work.

4. Connecting Links: What connected my triggers with the problem behavior?

Late to work. Got in trouble. Don't have money to get car fixed.

5. Problem Behavior Link: What was the problem behavior and any related behavior?

Went out at lunch, started drinking. Didn't return to work until the next day.

SOLUTION ANALYSIS WORKSHEET

Now it is time to explore each link to come up with more effective response strategies.

Vulnerability Link: <u>Everything seems to be going wrong.</u>

Solution #1: **<u>Turning the Mind</u>**

Solution #2: **<u>CARES</u>**

Solution #3: **<u>Be Mindful</u>**

Connecting Link: <u>Was up all night thinking about how much my life sucks.</u>

Solution #1: **<u>Turning the Mind</u>**

Solution #2: **<u>CARES</u>**

Solution #3: **<u>Be Mindful</u>**

Triggers Link: <u>Had to get a ride to work.</u>

Solution #1: **<u>CARES</u>**

Solution #2: **<u>DEAR WOMAN or MAN</u>**

Solution #3: **<u>Be Mindful</u>**

Connecting Link: <u>Late to work.</u>

Solution #1: **<u>CARES</u>**

Solution #2: **<u>Be Mindful</u>**

Problem Behavior Link: <u>Went out at lunch, started drinking. Didn't return to work until the next day.</u>

Solution #1: **<u>Turning the Mind</u>**

Solution #2: **<u>DEAR WOMAN or MAN</u>**

IN-DEPTH CHAIN ANALYSIS

What problem behavior are you analyzing?

 Wrote an angry letter to best friend ending relationship.

Now you are going to look at the chain of events that resulted in the problem behavior. These are referred to as links in the chain of events.

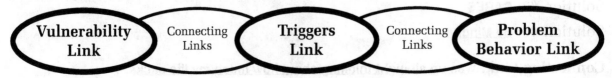

1. Vulnerability Link: In what ways was I vulnerable?

Worrying about being taken advantage of. Thinking that I can't trust people.

2. Connecting Links: What connected my vulnerability and triggers?

Obsessing with my thinking and keeping it all to myself.

3. Triggers Link: What were the internal, environmental, and interpersonal triggers?

My best friend didn't tell me that she was frustrated with me. She made plans without me.

4. Connecting Links: What connected my triggers with the problem behavior?

My best friend didn't answer her cell phone when I called. I was unable to reach any of my support system.

5. Problem Behavior Link: What was the problem behavior and any related behavior?

Wrote an angry letter to best friend saying that I couldn't trust her and would not be her friend anymore. Feel alone and hopeless. Wish my life was different.

SOLUTION ANALYSIS WORKSHEET

Now it is time to explore each link to come up with more effective response strategies.

Vulnerability Link: <u>**Thinking that I can't trust people.**</u>

Solution #1: <u>**Wise Mind**</u>

Solution #2: <u>**Effectively**</u>

Solution #3: <u>**Turtling**</u>

Connecting Link: <u>**Obsessing with my thinking.**</u>

Solution #1: <u>**Turtling**</u>

Solution #2: <u>**GIVE**</u>

Solution #3: <u>**Wise Mind**</u>

Triggers Link: <u>**Best friend didn't tell me that she was frustrated with me.**</u>

Solution #1: <u>**Effectively**</u>

Solution #2: <u>**Turtling**</u>

Solution #3: <u>**GIVE**</u>

Connecting Link: <u>**Unable to reach any of my support system.**</u>

Solution #1: <u>**Effectively**</u>

Solution #2: <u>**Turtling**</u>

Solution #3: <u>**FAST**</u>

Problem Behavior Link: <u>**Wrote an angry letter.**</u>

Solution #1: <u>**Turtling**</u>

Solution #2: <u>**GIVE**</u>

Solution #3: <u>**Wise Mind**</u>

PHONE CONSULTATION

This component of DBT provides clients with an opportunity to receive coaching in their day-to-day lives when they have problematic urges to hurt themselves or others or urges to damage their lives. This is an excellent way for clients to interrupt their destructive processes and replace these behaviors with more pro-social skills. This leads to clients being more effective in their lives.

Phone consultation is probably most useful with clients who over-utilize the acute care system. The client who has a tendency to go to the emergency room a lot or be hospitalized often can make use of phone consultation. Instead of creating crises clients can access their clinician or another designee who can coach them in using their skills. When clients use their skills they can avoid crises, self-harm, or suicide attempts.

Keep in mind that while phone consultation is useful for some clients it can foster dependence with others. These clients can seek advice from their clinician too often, leaving them hesitant about, or even incapable of, making decisions on their own.

An additional caveat with phone consultation is the burden it can place on the clinician. In the worst case scenario the clinician ends up spending most of his time, both at and away from work, on the phone with clients. This leaves the clinician out of balance with insufficient time and energy to take care of himself, to be invested in personal relationships, or to have fun or even downtime. Each clinician needs to decide when and how he might offer phone consultation to clients. It is possible to provide DBT treatment without offering phone consultation.

Alternatives to phone consultation include community support meetings, 12-step groups, sponsors, or mentors. There are obviously strengths and weaknesses of each resource and clinicians should work with their clients to determine the best options for each of them.

CONSULTATION TEAM

This is the equivalent of group supervision with a specific DBT structure (Linehan, 1993a; Linehand 1993b). The consultation provides support and accountability as a clinician discusses challenges with a client, complications in treatment, and countertransference. Team members can assist the clinician with remaining in balance and holding the dialectics by practicing DBT with him. Each DBT clinician uses the skills himself to stay connected to the work as well as to avoid negativity and burnout.

When a clinician is viewing a client judgmentally, or gets out of balance with positive or negative feelings, the treatment team helps the clinician to see situations and relationships from other perspectives. The treatment team supports the individual clinician and provides positive feedback. The treatment team also helps clinicians to be both active and passive to balance these two qualities and helps the clinician stay mindful of the dialectics covered in Chapter 2. The treatment team keeps all members grounded in imperfect consistency, enlightened self-interest, and interdependence with one another.

It is important to have healthy boundaries in treatment teams. A consultation team is group supervision, not group therapy. Clinicians' struggles, ups and downs, and successes are discussed as they relate to the clinical work. When the team begins to focus more on the clinician's life outside of therapeutic work it is time for the clinician to consider outside supervision or personal therapy.

There are six conditions to which DBT teams agree (Linehan 1993a; Linehan, 1993b):

- The philosophy of DBT: that clients are emotional dysregulated and in invalidating environments.

- Clinicians will consult with the client about how to design treatments and interact with other treatment professionals. The client is in the driver's seat. There are no closed-door meetings in which a client's fate is determined.

- Clinicians agree to be as consistent as possible; however, the other half of this dialectic is that consistency is imperfect even when at its best.

- All clinicians have limits. The treatment team supports clinicians observing their limits, asking for help, and rotating who takes the lead in difficult situations.

- Clinicians agree to remain non-judgmental with clients, family, self, the treatment team, and the system.

- Finally, the treatment team agrees that mistakes are made and everyone is fallible.

Consultation teams typically start with a mindfulness exercise, reviewing the six agreements by reading them aloud and then the agenda is collaboratively agreed upon. This consultation helps to maintain fidelity to DBT and to ensure that the hierarchy of behavior targets is triaged appropriately. DBT calls for issues to be addressed in the following order (Linehan, 1993a; Linehan, 1993b):

1. Life-threatening behavior

2. Therapy-interfering behavior

3. Behaviors that reduce quality of life

4. Increasing functioning through use of skills

5. Dealing with any trauma issues

6. Increasing respect for self

7. Working on individual goals

Because DBT clients are high-need, challenging clients who sometimes seem to get worse instead of better, it is essential that clinicians stay in balance, invest in the clients, and take care of themselves. A significant part of this process includes avoiding the Anti-DBT tactics outlined in Chapter 1.

As with phone consultation, it is possible to practice DBT without being in a formal consultation team. Clinicians are highly encouraged to have professional support and colleagues to interact with and to engage in formal supervision or consultation on an as-needed basis.

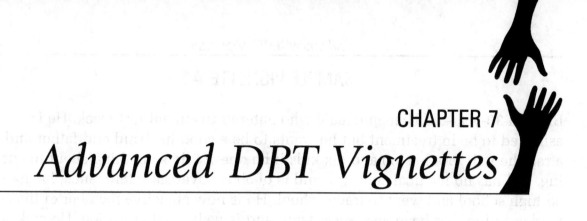

CHAPTER 7
Advanced DBT Vignettes

This chapter contains many opportunities to practice using DBT with clinical vignettes. There are ten categories of vignettes:

- Anger
- Anxiety
- Bipolar Disorders
- Conduct Disorder
- Depression
- Eating
- Impulse Control
- Substance Abuse
- Substance Dependence
- Trauma

There are three options in each of these categories. There is typically a clinical example of an adult and a youth displaying problems in that category. Not all of the vignettes will reflect clients seen by clinicians reading this text. There is space after each vignette for additional data. This section is designed for clinicians to delete, add, and revise the vignette so that it more closely matches clients served by the clinician. There is also a blank box so clinicians can explore one of their clients in that category. Just as the skills have to be relevant to the clients, these practice exercises need to be relevant to the clinician. Don't get caught up in the content of the vignettes. Adjust them so that they are reflective of your practice. It's the process of these practice exercises that is important. It is about thinking through how each clinician would use DBT skills with different clients.

There are two examples of how to complete the vignettes. After conceptualizing the vignette the clinician picks two skills from each of the four DBT categories. The clinician then writes down what skills they would teach the client and how they would teach the skills to the clients. This is a bit of a parallel process to how clients learn the skills. By thinking it through, making it relevant to their practice, and overcoming any fears or doubts, clinicians are considerably more likely to integrate DBT skills into their clinical practice.

SAMPLE VIGNETTE #1

Bill is a 30-year-old Hispanic male who entered treatment last week. He is ashamed to be in treatment but he wants to be a good husband and father and is afraid he will lose his job and his kids if he doesn't do something about his drinking. Bill has no medical concerns and is of above-average intelligence; he graduated high school and went to trade school. He is now an active member of the steelworker union, has been very successful, and is well liked at his job. He makes more than $50,000 a year and owns a home.

Bill normally drinks until he passes out on the weekends, but completed detox 10 days ago and hasn't had a drink since then, although he reports that he smokes pot most days. He seems to understand that he drinks and smokes to manage his moods. He was in recovery before for about a year when he was 25 years-old, and his two stays in residential treatment and three cycles of outpatient services have used all his insurance so he has to pay for treatment out of pocket.

Bill is quite depressed and worries that things won't improve no matter what he does. He reports having low energy and having been pessimistic about life for about 10 years. He is not suicidal nor does he have any psychotic symptoms but he believes he has nothing to offer his kids or his employer. His family knows he can lead a happier life. He has lost track of his religious community. Bill states that all his Latino friends drink and use and wonders why it isn't a problem for them. He gets embarrassed when he says he isn't as much of a man as his friends because he can't control it.

DBT SKILLS

In each skills area pick two skills that you would teach this client. Why these skills? How would you teach them? Adapt skills to be developmentally appropriate and culturally responsive.

MINDFULNESS:

1. **Wise Mind:** I think Bill would benefit from being in balance, and will act in his own best interest more often if he is in his Wise Mind. I would teach this skill by defining the skill and sharing an example or two of being in Wise Mind. Then I would ask Bill to think of a time that he was in Wise Mind and have him role-play the situation. We would discuss barriers and obstacles to being in Wise Mind, and how to overcome those barriers. I would then assign him to be in Wise Mind as much as possible.

2. **Participation:** Using examples from his life, I would explore times when Bill has participated fully in his life. I'd ask him how that has been useful and how it has not been useful. Then I would ask him to think about times when his participation in a situation or interaction was minimal, and ask him to evaluate how that went well and how it didn't. This exercise would

illustrate that participation would be more effective for him. I would also ask him how he can be more effective in his life, then give him the assignment to participate as much as possible in his life until we meet again.

DISTRESS TOLERANCE:

3. **Keeping it in Perspective:** I think it would help Bill to realize that he has gotten through a lot in his life and that he can get through this too. I would ask him to think about other times he didn't think he could accomplish a task or be successful, but in the end he was. I would use the metaphor that this is the marathon of stressful situations. All of the other stress that he has encountered up till now has been in training, so he is in the best shape of his life to handle this situation.

4. **Crisis Survival Network:** Bill should have a support system that will empower him to be the Latino man that he wants to be, in a productive and pro-social manner. Community supports and connection to religious communities might be very useful for him. I would ask him to come to the next session with at least three potential supporters on his list and details about how he could use them.

EMOTIONAL REGULATION:

5. **Ride the Emotion:** I want to help Bill to know that he can get through this. He can ride the difficult emotions and become stronger and more effective by doing so. When it gets tough or stressful, all he has to do is ride the emotion and impulse without having to take actions that would make it worse. One way to use this skill in session is to imagine actually surfing the emotions or impulses. I would assign him to practice this in his life between now and the next session.

6. **Radical Acceptance:** I think Bill would benefit from learning what he can control: his thoughts, feelings, and actions. In addition it would be useful for him to realize that there are many things that he can't control. I would practice focusing his attention and energy on what he can control and letting go of, or ignoring, the things he can't control. I would tie this idea to a cultural or religious value if related. I would ask him to take at least 3–5 minutes to practice Radical Acceptance each day until the next meeting.

INTERPERSONAL EFFECTIVENESS:

7. **Relationship Assumptions:** These would help Bill better manage his relationships. I would practice using these assumptions in session by reframing the way he is talking about things. I would ask him to dedicate time and energy to applying this to his life between sessions.

8. **Four Horsemen:** This metaphor would speak to Bill because of his connection to the Catholic Church. It would be a useful exercise to have him identify how bringing any or all of these into his relationships has been destructive in the past. I would have him role-play how to avoid these, while effectively dealing with frustrations and I would ask him to watch for the horsemen in the next week and think about how he can effectively combat them.

SAMPLE VIGNETTE #2

Rachel is a 13-year-old female who has been referred to treatment by Child Protective Services after years of emotional and physical abuse by both her parents. During Rachel's elementary school years, her parents manufactured and sold meth out of their home. She spent a year in foster care and has been adopted by her maternal aunt and uncle, who have three other daughters. They appear to be good parents and provide a nice home for Rachel. She seems to be adjusting reasonably well, although she has had some problems in school with aggressive and intimidating behavior. You worry about her potential to start using drugs since she uses slang that refers to drug use and seems to see it as a normal activity in which people typically engage. You are also concerned about her engaging in sexual behavior. She tells you that she participated in oral sex with boys at her old school. She wears long sleeves and dresses in black. You suspect that she engages in self-harm behavior, but don't know that directly. If she isn't doing this, she is certainly at risk for developing the behavior in the future.

DBT SKILLS

In each of the skills areas, pick two skills that you would teach this client. Why these skills? How would you teach them?

MINDFULNESS:

1. **Non-judgmental:** This will be enormously empowering to Rachel. I would start by defining non-judgmental and contrast it with judgmental thoughts, feelings, and actions. I'd ask her about when she feels judged by others and then ask her about times when she has judged others. Finally, I would ask her how she judges herself. My goal would be to educate her that judgments make things worse than they need to be. I would give her permission to not like things or to be unhappy, but with the knowledge that she doesn't have to view herself or others negatively. I would help her identify a self-judgment and then have her imagine setting it free or letting it go. Then I would ask her to remind herself to let go of this judgment in the morning and evening every day until we meet again. I would challenge her to not judge herself about how well she does.

2. **Turtling:** I would teach Rachel about the five ways that turtles take care of themselves, and ask her to think about how each of these ways would be useful for her. Then I would ask her to utilize all these ways between now and the next session. Before ending, I would make sure to discuss barriers and obstacles to turtling in her life and how to overcome those barriers.

DISTRESS TOLERANCE:

3. **Half-Smile:** This would be a useful skill for Rachel because it would help her to get in balance. I would help her find something to have a half-smile about right now. Then I would ask her to think of something stressful or difficult in her life recently, then to have a half smile on her face even while dealing with this stressor or difficulty. I would then ask her to set her alarm for one time a day that she can practice having a half-smile.

4. **Turning the Mind:** This skill would tap into Rachel's desire to be an adult, by talking about how she can drive her thoughts. I would use art work or visualization to express this.

EMOTIONAL REGULATION:

5. **ABC:** I would teach her this acronym and talk about how it might be useful, then I would have her think of situations in which it would be useful as well as some in which it would be hard, then have her role-play an example for each perspective. I would ask her if she knows anyone who does something like this well, then I'd ask her to interview that person and report back.

6. **Love Dandelions:** I would explain that this skill is about accepting the positives and negatives about ourselves. I would use art work for her to draw herself as a dandelion, and have her look at how it is attractive and not attractive. We would talk about how dandelions are resilient and great at surviving, just like she is. Then I'd ask her to use this skill with herself and others as much as possible between this week and next.

INTERPERSONAL EFFECTIVENESS:

7. **DEAR WOMAN:** This would be a great skill for Rachel to be able to use with family, friends, and at school. I would teach her the acronym and then role-play, using it in several different situations. I would ask her when this would be hard for her to do, and then have her problem-solve how to use it anyway.

8. **Making Repairs:** I would discuss the ability to apologize when it is appropriate, how to accept an apology when it makes sense, and how to stay engaged in relationship even when we feel like running away. I would tie

this skill to a goal of hers to have good friendships, and educate her about how we have to take care of ourselves in relationships and behave in a manner consistent with our ethics and values. I would use a difficulty or conflict in my relationship with her to show how making repairs has allowed us to be closer, better understand each other, and address deeper issues.

ANGER VIGNETTE #1

John is a 41-year-old divorced white male who is mandated to treatment because of domestic violence. He has a live-in girlfriend and no children. He also reports that he throws bottles and puts his fists through walls. The police have been at his house at least three times in the past year. He has been unemployed for more than a year, and reports being fired because of his outbursts and inability to work with others. He tried to start his own business, but couldn't seem to get along with potential customers, and has been living off of a small inheritance. He has some loyal friends who help take care of him when he can't buy groceries. He and his girlfriend talk about wanting to make their relationship work. John displays a sense of humor and motivation to do things differently.

Additional client data: _____

_____

_____

_____

DBT SKILLS

In each of the skills areas, pick two skills that you would teach this client. Why these skills? How would you teach them?

MINDFULNESS:

1. _____

_____

_____

2. _____

_____

_____

DISTRESS TOLERANCE:

3. _____

   _____

   _____

4. _____

   _____

   _____

EMOTIONAL REGULATION:

5. _____

   _____

   _____

6. _____

   _____

   _____

INTERPERSONAL EFFECTIVENESS:

7. _____

   _____

   _____

   _____

8. _____

   _____

   _____

ANGER VIGNETTE #2

Carrie is a 19-year-old Asian American with significant anger problems. She has come into therapy because she loses control of her anger. She finds her own behavior very embarrassing and feels that she brings shame to her family. She gets very upset at her co-workers and neighbors. She describes her anger as "coming out of nowhere." She yells, uses obscenities and stomps out of the room. She is not sure why she behaves this way. She reports wanting to go to college, but had to go to work to support her parents and grandparents, and she now spends most of her free time taking care of her grandparents. She says that she had one boyfriend in high school, but her family disapproved because he was African American. She judges herself as not deserving to have anything good in her life. This problem has been going on for the last 2 years.

Additional client data: _____

_____

_____

_____

DBT SKILLS

In each of the skills areas, pick two skills that you would teach this client. Why these skills? How would you teach them?

MINDFULNESS:

1. _____

_____

_____

2. _____

_____

_____

DISTRESS TOLERANCE:

3. _____

_____

_____

4. _____

_____

_____

EMOTIONAL REGULATION:

5. _____

_____

_____

6. _____

_____

_____

INTERPERSONAL EFFECTIVENESS:

7. _____

_____

_____

8. _____

_____

_____

ANGER VIGNETTE #3

Client details:

DBT SKILLS

In each of the skills areas, pick two skills that you would teach this client. Why these skills? How would you teach them?

MINDFULNESS:

1. _____

_____

_____

2. _____

_____

_____

DISTRESS TOLERANCE:

3. _____

   _____

4. _____

   _____

   _____

EMOTIONAL REGULATION:

5. _____

   _____

6. _____

   _____

   _____

INTERPERSONAL EFFECTIVENESS:

7. _____

   _____

   _____

8. _____

   _____

   _____

ANXIETY VIGNETTE #1

Brian is a 39-year-old Native American male. He reports coming into treatment because he is very concerned that his life is out of control. He reports having the same thoughts over and over again. He engages in rituals in order to be able to leave his house or his work. It takes him more than two hours to leave and commute, even though he only lives five miles from work. He has no social support. Because of his rituals and concerns, he does nothing except work, has no recreational activities or interests.

Additional client data: _____

_____

_____

_____

DBT SKILLS

In each of the skills areas, pick two skills that you would teach this client. Why these skills? How would you teach them?

MINDFULNESS:

1. _____

_____

_____

2. _____

_____

_____

DISTRESS TOLERANCE:

3. _____

   _____

   _____

4. _____

   _____

   _____

EMOTIONAL REGULATION:

5. _____

   _____

   _____

6. _____

   _____

   _____

INTERPERSONAL EFFECTIVENESS:

7. _____

   _____

   _____

   _____

8. _____

   _____

   _____

ANXIETY VIGNETTE #2

Pam is a 16-year-old Asian female. She has been coming to see you for three months. She is often late because she can't seem to get out of the house on time. She states that she is worried about leaving her house. She is fearful about being embarrassed or not being able to get out of the classroom if there is a problem. She takes Ativan several times a day to cope with this. This has been going on for about a year. She worries that she has missed so much school she won't graduate. Although she is very bright and thinks about a career, she can't imagine going to college.

Additional client data: _____

_____

_____

_____

DBT SKILLS

In each of the skills areas, pick two skills that you would teach this client. Why these skills? How would you teach them?

MINDFULNESS:

1. _____

_____

_____

2. _____

_____

_____

DISTRESS TOLERANCE:

3. _____

_____

_____

4. _____

_____

_____

EMOTIONAL REGULATION:

5. _____

_____

_____

6. _____

_____

_____

INTERPERSONAL EFFECTIVENESS:

7. _____

_____

_____

8. _____

_____

_____

ANXIETY VIGNETTE #3

Client details:

DBT SKILLS

In each of the skills areas, pick two skills that you would teach this client. Why these skills? How would you teach them?

MINDFULNESS:

1. _____

_____

_____

2. _____

_____

_____

DISTRESS TOLERANCE:

3. _____

   _____

   _____

4. _____

   _____

   _____

EMOTIONAL REGULATION:

5. _____

   _____

   _____

6. _____

   _____

   _____

INTERPERSONAL EFFECTIVENESS:

7. _____

   _____

   _____

8. _____

   _____

   _____

BIPOLAR VIGNETTE #1

Larry is a 19-year-old African American male with a history of depression. He has never been hospitalized for mental health problems or been psychotic. He also experiences elevated moods and extreme excitement about life. During these times, he goes from sleeping 8–10 hours to 3–4 hours a night. He reports this is a time of high creativity, as well as excessive spending and being very social. One of his major hobbies is listening to and playing music. He feels that he does this particularly well when he feels "up." He states that life is great when he is "up." If only he could be "up" all of the time.

Additional client data: _____

_____

_____

_____

DBT SKILLS

In each of the skills areas, pick two skills that you would teach this client. Why these skills? How would you teach them?

MINDFULNESS:

1. _____

_____

_____

2. _____

_____

_____

DISTRESS TOLERANCE:

3. _____

_____

_____

4. _____

_____

_____

EMOTIONAL REGULATION:

5. _____

_____

_____

6. _____

_____

_____

INTERPERSONAL EFFECTIVENESS:

7. _____

_____

_____

_____

8. _____

_____

_____

_____

BIPOLAR VIGNETTE #2

Julie is a 50-year-old divorced white female who lives alone. She has three grown children whom she sees on a regular basis. She has worked as an elementary school teacher for more than 20 years, and has a family history of depression. She has been in the hospital several times for psychotic behavior, during which she gets extremely sexual, and appears to be pleasure-seeking. Her mood becomes irritable; her speech is pressured and doesn't always make sense, even though she is not intoxicated. She is worried about using Meth to keep her "mania" going. Julie knows that taking care of herself helps to keep her stable, but she does so much for others, she doesn't have any energy left.

Additional client data: _____

_____

_____

_____

DBT SKILLS

In each of the skills areas, pick two skills that you would teach this client. Why these skills? How would you teach them?

MINDFULNESS:

1. _____

_____

_____

2. _____

_____

_____

DISTRESS TOLERANCE:

3. _____

_____

_____

4. _____

_____

_____

EMOTIONAL REGULATION:

5. _____

_____

_____

6. _____

_____

INTERPERSONAL EFFECTIVENESS:

7. _____

_____

_____

8. _____

_____

_____

BIPOLAR VIGNETTE #3

Client details:

DBT SKILLS

In each of the skills areas, pick two skills that you would teach this client. Why these skills? How would you teach them?

MINDFULNESS:

1. _____

_____

_____

2. _____

_____

_____

DISTRESS TOLERANCE:

3. _____

_____

_____

4. _____

_____

_____

EMOTIONAL REGULATION:

5. _____

_____

_____

6. _____

_____

_____

INTERPERSONAL EFFECTIVENESS:

7. _____

_____

_____

8. _____

_____

_____

CONDUCT/OPPOSITIONAL DEFIANT VIGNETTE #1

Sheri is a 15-year-old white female who has been in treatment with you for the last 6 months. She has an explosive temper; she breaks things, and harms others. She does well in school, but was diagnosed with conduct disorder when she was younger because of fire-setting and harm done to animals. She feels that others are around to help her achieve her goals, and is not concerned about others' feelings. She buys drugs for her friends so that they will help her get even with others. She has been involved with juvenile justice on a number of occasions. She lives with her parents and a younger brother. The parents are very busy with their careers and Sheri often finds herself babysitting and making dinner for herself and her brother.

Additional client data: _____

_____

_____

DBT SKILLS

In each of the skills areas, pick two skills that you would teach this client. Why these skills? How would you teach them?

MINDFULNESS:

1. _____

_____

_____

2. _____

_____

_____

DISTRESS TOLERANCE:

3. _____

_____

_____

4. _____

_____

_____

EMOTIONAL REGULATION:

5. _____

_____

_____

6. _____

_____

_____

INTERPERSONAL EFFECTIVENESS:

7. _____

_____

_____

_____

8. _____

_____

_____

_____

CONDUCT/OPPOSITIONAL DEFIANT VIGNETTE #2

Adam is a 22-year-old Latino male. He recently graduated college, although this was his third school. He had been kicked out of two previous colleges for property damage and hazing other students. He lives at home with his widowed mother. He reports that he has no intention of getting a job or moving out, since his mother is happy to take care of him. Adam hangs out with individuals with criminal backgrounds. He may have engaged in identity theft. He doesn't seem to care how other people live their lives. He states that should be able to take it easy for the rest of his life. He is not going to be one of those people living in the suburbs paying the bank a bunch of money.

Additional client data: _____

_____

_____

_____

DBT SKILLS

In each of the skills areas, pick two skills that you would teach this client. Why these skills? How would you teach them?

MINDFULNESS:

1. _____

_____

_____

2. _____

_____

_____

DISTRESS TOLERANCE:

3. _____

_____

_____

4. _____

_____

_____

EMOTIONAL REGULATION:

5. _____

_____

_____

6. _____

_____

_____

INTERPERSONAL EFFECTIVENESS:

7. _____

_____

_____

8. _____

_____

_____

CONDUCT/OPPOSITIONAL DEFIANT VIGNETTE #3

Client details:

DBT SKILLS

In each of the skills areas, pick two skills that you would teach this client. Why these skills? How would you teach them?

MINDFULNESS:

1. _____

   _____

   _____

2. _____

   _____

   _____

   _____

DISTRESS TOLERANCE:

3. _____

   _____

   _____

4. _____

   _____

   _____

EMOTIONAL REGULATION:

5. _____

   _____

   _____

6. _____

   _____

   _____

INTERPERSONAL EFFECTIVENESS:

7. _____

   _____

   _____

   _____

8. _____

   _____

   _____

   _____

DEPRESSION VIGNETTE #1

George is a 16-year-old African American male. He comes into treatment because he got kicked out of his parents' house, and he has been living on the streets for the last 6 months. He dropped out of high school. He reports not having the energy to get a job, and states that all he wants to do is sleep all the time. He wants to live a life like he sees on TV, but he feels like a failure. Why did this have to happen to him, he wonders. He has very few friends and can't contact any of his extended family because he can't face how his life has turned out. He reports really wanting his life to get better.

Additional client data: _____

_____

_____

_____

DBT SKILLS

In each of the skills areas, pick two skills that you would teach this client. Why these skills? How would you teach them?

MINDFULNESS:

1. _____

_____

_____

2. _____

_____

_____

DISTRESS TOLERANCE:

3. _____

   _____

   _____

4. _____

   _____

   _____

EMOTIONAL REGULATION:

5. _____

   _____

   _____

6. _____

   _____

   _____

INTERPERSONAL EFFECTIVENESS:

7. _____

   _____

   _____

8. _____

   _____

   _____

DEPRESSION VIGNETTE #2

Sally enters treatment with you. She is a 36-year-old bicultural female who has been married for twelve years. She has been using pain pills to get through the days since her twins were born three months ago. She reports having used alcohol and pot in college, but not in the last five years. She reports never getting any rest and being tired all of the time. She is not suicidal and you are not concerned. She is worried about money and how she is going to keep the house going with this third and fourth child. They will have to move soon, since they are in a one-bedroom apartment. Her husband is supportive, but is at work most of the time. They moved here from the East Coast, so they have no family or friends to support them locally.

Additional client data: _____

_____

_____

_____

DBT SKILLS

In each of the skills areas, pick two skills that you would teach this client. Why these skills? How would you teach them?

MINDFULNESS:

1. _____

_____

_____

2. _____

_____

_____

DISTRESS TOLERANCE:

3. _____

_____

_____

4. _____

_____

_____

EMOTIONAL REGULATION:

5. _____

_____

_____

6. _____

_____

_____

INTERPERSONAL EFFECTIVENESS:

7. _____

_____

_____

8. _____

_____

_____

DEPRESSION VIGNETTE #3

Client details:

DBT SKILLS

In each of the skills areas, pick two skills that you would teach this client. Why these skills? How would you teach them?

MINDFULNESS:

1. _____

_____

_____

2. _____

_____

_____

DISTRESS TOLERANCE:

3. _____

   _____

   _____

4. _____

   _____

   _____

EMOTIONAL REGULATION:

5. _____

   _____

   _____

6. _____

   _____

   _____

INTERPERSONAL EFFECTIVENESS:

7. _____

   _____

   _____

   _____

8. _____

   _____

   _____

EATING VIGNETTE #1

Tammy is a 13-year-old white female, about average weight for her height, who binges and then throws up. She reports being always hungry and then very upset after she eats. She figures that she can eat as much as see wants and then vomit and never gain any weight. She has recently started exercising, in which she engages for one to two hours a day. She hates herself and she hates her family, all of whom are significantly overweight. She says she is going to graduate high school and never look back. She is never going to be fat and lazy like her family.

Additional client data: _____

_____

_____

_____

DBT SKILLS

In each of the skills areas, pick two skills that you would teach this client. Why these skills? How would you teach them?

MINDFULNESS:

1. _____

_____

_____

2. _____

_____

_____

DISTRESS TOLERANCE:

3. _____

_____

_____

4. _____

_____

_____

EMOTIONAL REGULATION:

5. _____

_____

_____

6. _____

_____

_____

INTERPERSONAL EFFECTIVENESS:

7. _____

_____

_____

_____

8. _____

_____

_____

_____

EATING VIGNETTE #2

Boyd is a 28-year-old single white, openly gay male. He reports cruising the gym and the clubs a lot for romantic encounters. He states that it is essential to look healthy, so he eats less than 1200 calories a day. While he enjoys a good glass of wine, he doesn't allow himself the calories. If he does eat a full meal, he takes 50 or more laxatives. Boyd doesn't have any family support, since they don't support his lifestyle. Boyd was raised in a religious family. He reports having a lot of guilt and shame for not turning out to be more normal.

Additional client data: _____

_____

_____

_____

DBT SKILLS

In each of the skills areas, pick two skills that you would teach this client. Why these skills? How would you teach them?

MINDFULNESS:

1. _____

_____

_____

2. _____

_____

_____

DISTRESS TOLERANCE:

3. _____

   _____

   _____

4. _____

   _____

   _____

EMOTIONAL REGULATION:

5. _____

   _____

   _____

6. _____

   _____

INTERPERSONAL EFFECTIVENESS:

7. _____

   _____

   _____

8. _____

   _____

   _____

EATING VIGNETTE #3

Client details:

DBT SKILLS

In each of the skills areas, pick two skills that you would teach this client. Why these skills? How would you teach them?

MINDFULNESS:

1. _____

_____

_____

2. _____

_____

_____

DISTRESS TOLERANCE:

3. _____

_____

_____

4. _____

_____

_____

EMOTIONAL REGULATION:

5. _____

_____

_____

6. _____

_____

_____

INTERPERSONAL EFFECTIVENESS:

7. _____

_____

_____

8. _____

_____

_____

IMPULSE CONTROL ISSUES VIGNETTE #1

Mary is a 16-year-old African American female, brought into treatment by her parents. They are worried about her because they found marijuana in her room. She also got a "Minor in Possession" while attending a large party at a friend's house. She self-identifies as a "party girl." Mary doesn't think she needs to be in treatment; she isn't crazy, just a normal teenager. She states that everyone is playing "Jackass" games, but she isn't going to get hurt because she is too cool. Both her older sisters had babies before the age of 20. Mary has run away twice in the last 18 months. She is dressed seductively and appears to be underweight. Her parents are very concerned about how quickly she engages in out-of-control behavior.

Additional client data: _____

_____

_____

_____

DBT SKILLS

In each of the skills areas, pick two skills that you would teach this client. Why these skills? How would you teach them?

MINDFULNESS:

1. _____

_____

_____

2. _____

_____

_____

DISTRESS TOLERANCE:

3. _____

_____

_____

4. _____

_____

_____

EMOTIONAL REGULATION:

5. _____

_____

_____

6. _____

_____

_____

INTERPERSONAL EFFECTIVENESS:

7. _____

_____

_____

8. _____

_____

_____

IMPULSE CONTROL ISSUES VIGNETTE #2

Charlie, a 47-year-old Asian male, comes into treatment because he keeps "screwing up his life." He tends to quit jobs very suddenly, and reports not completing projects and tasks on a regular basis. He has lost a lot of money gambling. Charlie reports jumping from one romantic relationship to another, and says his parents gave up years ago on his getting married and having children. He says he is ashamed of not being the son his parents wanted. He feels like a big failure, and has very little hope that his life can be different.

Additional client data: _____

_____

_____

_____

DBT SKILLS

In each of the skills areas, pick two skills that you would teach this client. Why these skills? How would you teach them?

MINDFULNESS:

1. _____

_____

_____

2. _____

_____

_____

DISTRESS TOLERANCE:

3. _____

   _____

   _____

4. _____

   _____

   _____

EMOTIONAL REGULATION:

5. _____

   _____

   _____

6. _____

   _____

INTERPERSONAL EFFECTIVENESS:

7. _____

   _____

   _____

8. _____

   _____

   _____

IMPULSE CONTROL ISSUES VIGNETTE #3

Client details:

DBT SKILLS

In each of the skills areas, pick two skills that you would teach this client. Why these skills? How would you teach them?

MINDFULNESS:

1. _____

_____

_____

2. _____

_____

_____

DISTRESS TOLERANCE:

3. _____

_____

_____

4. _____

_____

_____

EMOTIONAL REGULATION:

5. _____

_____

_____

_____

6. _____

_____

_____

INTERPERSONAL EFFECTIVENESS:

7. _____

_____

_____

_____

8. _____

_____

_____

_____

SUBSTANCE ABUSE VIGNETTE #1

Ralph, a 17-year-old bicultural sophomore in high school, was held back in seventh grade. He appears to be of average intelligence and has a great sense of humor. He also has ADD, and has a hard time behaving appropriately in the classroom. He has C+ average; however, you suspect he is bored and doesn't see any value in working harder academically. He recently got his driver's license and works part time at a fast-food place. He has a girlfriend who is 3 months pregnant. He feels like a failure, because his mother had him when she was 16, so he feels like he is repeating her mistakes. He wants to be a responsible father, since he never met his own father. He reports not sleeping because he is so worried about what he is going to do, and smoking pot to relax and get a break from all the stress. He also tells you that he is just being a typical teenager and should not have to be responsible in his life just yet. He doesn't think it is big deal to not do well in school, engage in sexual behavior, and use drugs.

Additional client data: _____

_____

_____

_____

DBT SKILLS

In each of the skills areas, pick two skills that you would teach this client. Why these skills? How would you teach them?

MINDFULNESS:

1. _____

_____

_____

2. _____

_____

_____

DISTRESS TOLERANCE:

3. _____

   _____

4. _____

   _____

EMOTIONAL REGULATION:

5. _____

   _____

   _____

6. _____

   _____

   _____

INTERPERSONAL EFFECTIVENESS:

7. _____

   _____

   _____

8. _____

   _____

   _____

SUBSTANCE ABUSE VIGNETTE #2

Rachel is a 33-year-old African American client who has been encouraged to see you by a friend who hopes she can stop getting high and deal with the pain in her life. She reports being a biological male, but psychologically a woman; she began living as woman the majority of time approximately 2 years ago. She confides in you that her being transgendered conflicts with her faith. She works full time and has a college degree. She wishes her life was easier and more normal; her siblings have married, have children, and own their own homes. Her family doesn't know she is transgendered. She talks about how they would be disappointed and her culture would reject her. She reports using Meth and marijuana, which get in the way of her work sometimes. She admits that she uses to forget about all the pain in her life. She also has been suicidal a number of times and has had a couple of hospitalizations.

Additional client data: _____

_____

_____

_____

DBT SKILLS

In each of the skills areas, pick two skills that you would teach this client. Why these skills? How would you teach them?

MINDFULNESS:

1. _____

_____

_____

2. _____

_____

_____

DISTRESS TOLERANCE:

3. _____

   _____

   _____

4. _____

   _____

   _____

EMOTIONAL REGULATION:

5. _____

   _____

   _____

6. _____

   _____

   _____

INTERPERSONAL EFFECTIVENESS:

7. _____

   _____

   _____

8. _____

   _____

   _____

SUBSTANCE ABUSE VIGNETTE #3

Client details:

DBT SKILLS

In each of the skills areas, pick two skills that you would teach this client. Why these skills? How would you teach them?

MINDFULNESS:

1. _____

_____

_____

2. _____

_____

_____

DISTRESS TOLERANCE:

3. _____

   _____

   _____

4. _____

   _____

   _____

EMOTIONAL REGULATION:

5. _____

   _____

   _____

6. _____

   _____

   _____

INTERPERSONAL EFFECTIVENESS:

7. _____

   _____

   _____

8. _____

   _____

   _____

SUBSTANCE DEPENDENCE VIGNETTE #1

Betty entered treatment last week. She completed detox 10 days ago, hasn't had a drink since then. A 25-year-old Native American female who is ashamed to be in treatment, she is afraid she'll lose her job and her kids if she doesn't do something about her drinking. On weekends, she drinks until she passes out. She reports that she smokes pot most days, and has been doing this since getting out of detox. She reports having had low energy and being pessimistic about life for about ten years. She is neither suicidal nor appears to have any psychotic symptoms. She doesn't feel that she has anything to offer her kids or at her job. She has had two DUIIs in the past and her family has expressed concerns about her being an inadequate parent.

Additional client data: _____

_____

_____

_____

DBT SKILLS

In each of the skills areas, pick two skills that you would teach this client. Why these skills? How would you teach them?

MINDFULNESS:

1. _____

_____

_____

2. _____

_____

_____

DISTRESS TOLERANCE:

3. _____

_____

_____

4. _____

_____

_____

EMOTIONAL REGULATION:

5. _____

_____

_____

_____

6. _____

_____

_____

INTERPERSONAL EFFECTIVENESS:

7. _____

_____

_____

_____

8. _____

_____

_____

SUBSTANCE DEPENDENCE VIGNETTE #2

Jake is a 14-year-old Latino male. He has been using Meth for the last two years and reports that he had his first drink at his First Communion ceremony when he was four years old. He comes across as cocky and uncaring. He states that he belongs to a gang, and says he won't live to age 25 with how poor his people are. He engages in risky behavior and has unprotected sex with different partners. He wants to go out in a blaze a glory, as opposed to working all his life for minimum wage. His parents were hoping that he would graduate high school and go to college.

Additional client data: _____

_____

_____

_____

DBT SKILLS

In each of the skills areas, pick two skills that you would teach this client. Why these skills? How would you teach them?

MINDFULNESS:

1. _____

_____

_____

2. _____

_____

_____

DISTRESS TOLERANCE:

3. _____

_____

_____

4. _____

_____

_____

EMOTIONAL REGULATION:

5. _____

_____

_____

6. _____

_____

_____

INTERPERSONAL EFFECTIVENESS:

7. _____

_____

_____

8. _____

_____

_____

SUBSTANCE DEPENDENCE VIGNETTE #3

Client details:

DBT SKILLS

In each of the skills areas, pick two skills that you would teach this client. Why these skills? How would you teach them?

MINDFULNESS:

1. _____

_____

_____

2. _____

_____

_____

DISTRESS TOLERANCE:

3. _____

_____

4. _____

_____

_____

EMOTIONAL REGULATION:

5. _____

_____

6. _____

_____

INTERPERSONAL EFFECTIVENESS:

7. _____

_____

_____

8. _____

_____

_____

TRAUMA VIGNETTE #1

Eric is a 55-year-old white male who came into treatment voluntarily, although he recently got a DUII, and who reports drinking daily since his wife left him. He says she left him due to their lack of intimacy and his oversensitivity, and he reports being beside himself. He startles easily, has memories that haunt him about living on the street and getting beaten up nearly every day. He has also done time in prison and you wonder if he was raped while he was there.

Additional client data: _____

_____

_____

_____

DBT SKILLS

In each of the skills areas, pick two skills that you would teach this client. Why these skills? How would you teach them?

MINDFULNESS:

1. _____

_____

_____

2. _____

_____

_____

DISTRESS TOLERANCE:

    3. _____

       _____

       _____

    4. _____

       _____

       _____

EMOTIONAL REGULATION:

    5. _____

       _____

       _____

    6. _____

       _____

       _____

INTERPERSONAL EFFECTIVENESS:

    7. _____

       _____

       _____

    8. _____

       _____

       _____

TRAUMA VIGNETTE #2

Lori is a 17-year-old bicultural female who is referred to treatment from Child Protective Services. She was sexually and physically abused by her father and uncle for more than a year. She protected her two younger sisters from being molested, although they did experience the physical abuse. Lori's mother died two years ago of lung cancer. Lori is emancipated and is her sisters' guardian. She wants to have a normal life, and is willing to do whatever it takes to be a functional adult and provide opportunities for her sisters. She states that if she continued to be the victim, her father would win and she won't let that happen.

Additional client data: _____

_____

_____

_____

DBT SKILLS

In each of the skills areas, pick two skills that you would teach this client. Why these skills? How would you teach them?

MINDFULNESS:

1. _____

_____

_____

2. _____

_____

_____

DISTRESS TOLERANCE:

3. _____

_____

_____

4. _____

_____

_____

EMOTIONAL REGULATION:

5. _____

_____

_____

6. _____

_____

_____

INTERPERSONAL EFFECTIVENESS:

7. _____

_____

_____

8. _____

_____

_____

TRAUMA VIGNETTE #3

Client details:

DBT SKILLS

In each of the skills areas, pick two skills that you would teach this client. Why these skills? How would you teach them?

MINDFULNESS:

1. _____

_____

_____

2. _____

_____

_____

DISTRESS TOLERANCE:

3. _____

_____

_____

4. _____

_____

_____

EMOTIONAL REGULATION:

5. _____

_____

_____

6. _____

_____

_____

INTERPERSONAL EFFECTIVENESS:

7. _____

_____

_____

8. _____

_____

_____

References

Hays, Pamela A. (2007). *Addressing Cultural Complexities in Practice: Assessment, Diagnosis, and Therapy: 2nd Edition.* APA: Washington, D.C.

Linehan, Marsha M. (1993a). *Cognitive-Behavioral Treatment of Borderline Personality Disorder.* Guilford Press: New York.

Linehan, Marsha M. (1993b). *Skills Training Manual for Treating Borderline Personality Disorder.* Guilford Press: New York.

Marra, Thomas, (2004). *Depressed & Anxious: The dialectical behavior therapy workbook for overcoming depression and anxiety.* New Harbinger Press: Oakland.

Marra, Thomas, (2005). *Dialectical Behavior Therapy in Private Practice: A practical and comprehensive guide.* New Harbinger Press: Oakland.

Miller, Alex L., Rathus, Jill H., Linehan, Marsha M. & Swensen, Charles R. (2006). *Dialectical Behavior Therapy with Suicidal Adolescents.* Guilford Press: New York.

Miller, William, & Rolnick, Stephen (2002). *Motivational Interviewing: 2nd edition.* Guilford Press: New York.

Moonshine, Cathy (2007). *Advanced Dialectical Behavior Therapy.* Eau Claire, WI: PESI. (Available at http://www.pesi.com)

Prochaska, James O., Norcross, John, & DiClemente, Carlo (1995). *Changing for Good: A Revolutionary Six-Stage Program for Overcoming Bad Habits and Moving Your Life Positively Forward.* Harper Collins: New York.

Spradlin, Scott E. (2003). *Don't let your emotions run your life: How dialectical behavior therapy can put you in control.* New Harbinger Press: Oakland.